Methadone Maintenance: A Physician's Guide to Treatment

Second Edition

Peter Selby, MBBS, CCFP
Meldon Kahan, MD, CCFP

camh
Centre for Addiction and Mental Health
Centre de toxicomanie et de santé mentale

Library and Archives Canada Cataloguing in Publication

Selby, Peter, 1965-

Methadone maintenance : a physician's guide to treatment / Peter Selby, Meldon Kahan. —2nd ed.

Includes bibliographical references.

Issued also in electronic format.

1. Methadone maintenance. I. Kahan, Meldon II. Centre for Addiction and Mental Health III. Title.

RC568.M4S45 2010 616.86'32061 C2009-906567-3

ISBN: 978-1-77052-892-5 (PRINT)
ISBN: 978-1-77052-893-2 (PDF)
ISBN: 978-1-77052-894-9 (HTML)
ISBN: 978-1-77052-895-6 (ePUB)

Printed in Canada

This publication may be available in other formats. For information about alternate formats or other CAMH publications, or to place an order, please contact Sales and Distribution:

Toll-free: 1 800 661-1111
Toronto: 416 595-6059
E-mail: publications@camh.net
Online store: http://store.camh.net

Website: www.camh.net

4266 / 3-2011 / PZ163

This manual was produced by the following:
Development: Andrew Johnson, CAMH
Editorial: Kelly Coleman; Nick Gamble, CAMH
Design: Nancy Leung, CAMH
Print production: Christine Harris, CAMH

Contents

Preface

Methadone maintenance has long been recognized as an effective treatment for opioid dependence. This guide is one of a series of professional resources that support physicians, pharmacists, counsellors and other health and social service professionals in providing methadone maintenance treatment.

Methadone Maintenance: A Physician's Guide to Treatment provides essential information on topics such as methadone dose tapering, drug interactions involving methadone, using methadone in opioid withdrawal management, managing pain in methadone-treated patients and managing pregnancy in women who use opioids.

While improving the availability and accessibility of methadone treatment are important goals, maintaining a high standard of care is essential. It is hoped that this manual will help achieve this goal by facilitating the provision of high-quality methadone treatment to patients across Ontario.

Peter Selby, MBBS, CCFP
Meldon Kahan, MD, CCFP, FRCPC
CAMH, August 2010

An important note

Medicine is an evolving science. As new research and clinical experience broaden our knowledge, treatment and drug therapy may change. In developing this guide, the authors, editors and publishers have referred to sources that are believed to be reliable. The contents of this book are based on information available as of 2007. However, in view of the possibility of human error or changes in medical science, none of the authors, editors or publishers nor any other party who has been involved in the preparation or publication of this text warrants that the information herein is in every respect accurate or complete, and they are not responsible for any errors or omissions or for the results obtained from the use of such information.

Readers are encouraged to confirm the information contained herein with other sources. Readers are particularly advised to check the product information sheet included in the package of any drug product they plan to administer, to be certain that the information obtained from this text or any other reference material is accurate and that changes have not been made in the recommended dose or in the contraindications for administration. This is of particular importance in connection with new or infrequently used drugs.

About the authors

Dr. Peter Selby, MBBS, CCFP, MHSc, is the Clinical Director of the Addictions Program and Head of the Nicotine Dependence Clinic at the Centre for Addiction and Mental Health. He is also an Associate Professor in the Department of Family and Community Medicine, the Department of Psychiatry and the Dalla Lanna School of Public Health at the University of Toronto.

Dr. Meldon Kahan, MD, CCFP, FRCPC, is an Associate Professor and researcher in the Department of Family Medicine at the University of Toronto. He is also Medical Director of the Addiction Medicine Service at St. Joseph's Health Centre in Toronto, and an author and editor of two textbooks on addiction.

Contributors

MMT AND CONCURRENT PSYCHIATRIC DISORDERS

Charl Els, MB ChB, FC Psych, MMed Psych, ASAM, MRO
Addictions Specialist, University of Alberta Hospital; Clinical Assistant Professor, Department of Psychiatry, University of Alberta

MMT AND CONCURRENT MEDICAL DISORDERS

Curtis Handford, MD, CCFP, MHSc
Staff Physician, CAMH and Department of Family and Community Medicine, St. Michael's Hospital, Toronto; Assistant Professor, Department of Family and Community Medicine, University of Toronto

URINE DRUG SCREENING AND TOXICOLOGY

Bhushan M. Kapur, D.Phil., C.Chem., FRSC, FACB, FCACB
Assistant Professor, Department of Laboratory Medicine and Pathobiology, Faculty of Medicine, University of Toronto; Scientist and consultant in toxicology, Division of Clinical Pharmacology and Toxicology, The Hospital for Sick Children, Toronto, and Department of Clinical Pathology, Sunnybrook Health Sciences Centre, Toronto.

PREGNANCY AND OPIOID USE

Alice Ordean, MD, CCFP, MHSc
Medical Director of the Toronto Centre for Substance Use in Pregnancy (T-CUP) at St. Joseph's Health Centre, Toronto; Assistant Professor, Department of Family and Community Medicine, University of Toronto

METHADONE OVERDOSE PROTOCOL

Anita Srivastava, MD, CCFP, MSc

This second edition of *Methadone Maintenance: A Physician's Guide to Treatment* is based on an edition originally published in 1998. The first edition was edited by Bruna Brands, PhD, and John Brands, MHSc.

The following individuals should also be acknowledged as many of their contributions, although revised and updated, are still reflected in this second edition: Michael Anderson, MLT, BSc; David Marsh, MD; Shelley McMain, PhD; Wayne Skinner, MSW, RSW; Neal Sutton, MD, LLB; and Lynn Wilson, MD.

SECTION I

Fundamental concepts in methadone maintenance treatment

CHAPTER 1

Fundamental clinical concepts in addiction medicine

This chapter begins with some definitions and background information on important concepts related to addictions, including physical dependence, tolerance and withdrawal. It also presents the diagnostic criteria for both substance dependence and substance abuse from the *Diagnostic and Statistical Manual of Disorders, 4th Edition* (DSM-IV), published by the American Psychiatric Association (APA). The chapter then summarizes the major theories of addiction and concludes with a brief overview of addiction treatment in general.

Key concepts of addiction

Before prescribing methadone for the treatment of opioid dependence, the prescribing physician needs to have a working knowledge of key concepts in addiction and a familiarity with the diagnostic criteria, in order to better understand patients who present for treatment.

ADDICTION

Addiction is a primary, chronic, neurobiological disease with genetic, psychosocial and environmental factors that influence its development and manifestations. It is characterized by behaviours that include one or more of the following:

- impaired control over drug use
- continued use despite harm
- compulsive use
- craving.

Typical comments from people with addictions regarding these "four Cs" are presented in Table 1-1.

TABLE 1-1

The four Cs of addiction

FEATURE	TYPICAL COMMENT
Loss of **control** over use	"Every time I try to limit my use to only once a week, I end up using every day." "I try to limit myself to one drink per day but once I start, I can't seem to stop till I pass out."
Continued use despite knowledge of harmful **consequences**	"I know my drug use caused my HIV but I can't stop using." "I have to stop using because my life is out of control, but using is the only option for me."

Continued on next page

TABLE 1-1: THE FOUR CS OF ADDICTION (continued)

FEATURE	TYPICAL COMMENT
Compulsion to use	"All I do is think about how I am going to score." "No matter what I do, I can't get drugs out of my mind and I feel I have to use and use a lot. Once I want to use, it is like I am on autopilot and I just have to use. I'll do anything to get drugs."
Craving	"It's like a physical drive or urge to use. I want it from the pit of my stomach, I get sweaty just thinking about it. At times, these urges come out of nowhere or I get them when I meet my using buddies, pass the corner where my dealer hangs out or when I am feeling down."

(Based on ASAM, 2003.)

PHYSICAL DEPENDENCE

Physical dependence is often thought to be the thing that defines addiction, but it is not always necessary or sufficient for a diagnosis of substance dependence, and modern definitions of addiction (such as the one presented above) de-emphasize its role. Nevertheless, understanding the components of physical dependence is important because they must be managed clinically with discontinuation of opioids. Physical dependence comprises two related observable phenomena: tolerance and withdrawal.

Tolerance

Tolerance results from compensatory changes, such as downregulation and desensitization, in the number and sensitivity of central nervous system (CNS) receptors. Over time, these changes compel patients to take more of the drug to achieve the same effect; if they maintain the same level and pattern of consumption, they stop experiencing the desired effect. The time it takes to develop tolerance differs considerably among the various effects of drugs of abuse. With opioids, tolerance to the analgesic effects develops slowly, whereas tolerance to the mood-altering effects (the "high") begins within days, leading some patients to "chase the high" by using increasing amounts. Tolerance to the respiratory-depressant effects of opioids takes months to develop and is never complete. Therefore, people who are dependent on opioids are always at risk of developing symptoms of overdose if they increase their amounts of opioids suddenly, or if the purity of their opioid suddenly increases and they use their usual amount.

Withdrawal

Withdrawal is a specific syndrome that often begins within a few hours of stopping the drug. It occurs because the downregulation of receptors (a process by which a cell decreases the number of receptors to a given hormone or neurotransmitter in order to reduce its sensitivity to it) leads to unstable neurotransmission. These receptors take days or weeks to normalize with abstinence, creating a constellation of symptoms and signs that are opposite to the drug's main effect.

The acute withdrawal for most drugs starts within a half-life of the drug, peaks within three to five half-lives and then resolves within a week or two at most. However, this period is often followed by intense cravings for the drug, dysphoric mood and other symptoms that can lead to relapse. Some experts call these symptoms "subacute withdrawal," although this concept has not been well defined scientifically. Relapse within the first few weeks of stopping the drug is generally attributable to poorly managed withdrawal. Therefore, most programs require that withdrawal be treated appropriately before the intensive phase of treatment begins. Methadone treatment, however, is an exception, requiring no prolonged period of withdrawal management before the first dose of methadone is administered.

SUBSTANCE-RELATED DISORDERS

Substance use disorders are listed under Axis I of the DSM-IV. This means that they meet the criteria for a disease, with a description of its onset, duration and prognosis, and that they have an associated treatment. Substance-related disorders are classified as either substance use disorders (which are further categorized as either substance abuse or substance dependence) or substance-induced disorders (such as cocaine-induced psychosis).

Substance abuse is a distinct disorder that almost always precedes the diagnosis of substance dependence. Once a patient meets the criteria for substance dependence, he or she can never meet the criteria for substance abuse for the same substance. However, not all patients who meet the criteria for substance abuse develop dependence.

Criteria for both disorders as listed in the DSM-IV are provided in Table 1-2 on page 6.

Theories of addiction

There are several theories of addiction, but the most compelling one views it as a multifactor disease caused by predisposing and precipitating factors (Volkow & Li, 2005). This theory describes the disease as the interaction between a host (the addict), an agent (the drug) and environmental determinants (such as social determinants of health), affected by a vector (e.g., a drug pusher or the tobacco industry) that promotes the drug and/or creates conducive conditions for its increased use and the subsequent harm associated with that use (Volkow, 2005).

There is emerging evidence that the neurobiology of addiction is the key to understanding why patients have great difficulty remaining abstinent, even years after withdrawal is overcome (Hyman & Malenka, 2001; Hyman, Malenka et al., 2006; Hyman, 2005). Briefly, the ventral tegmental area, the median forebrain bundle and the nucleus accumbens all constitute part of the mesolimbic dopaminergic system involved in the reward mechanisms of drugs of abuse. This system accounts for drug seeking, drug liking and drug wanting. Other structures, such as the mammillary bodies in the limbic system, are involved in long-term memory of the rewarding aspects of drugs of abuse. It appears that the brain is unable to differentiate between natural and unnatural reward, making it hard for the substance-dependent patient to stop compulsive use (Kalivas & Volkow, 2005).

HOST FACTORS

It is now evident that a large number of genetic factors play a role in predisposing some individuals to develop a substance use disorder when they experiment with drugs of abuse or are prescribed drugs for a condition such as anxiety or pain (Lachman, 2006). Other host factors include some personality traits (such as novelty seeking) and co-occurring psychiatric disorders.

DRUG FACTORS

Drugs that have abuse liability (i.e., are capable of being abused) are those that cross the blood-brain barrier and have the ability to release dopamine in the mesolimbic system. The abuse liability of a drug depends on several factors: its lipophilicity (i.e., the rate at which it enters into the CNS), its route of administration (inhaled drugs enter the CNS more rapidly than intravenous ones, which in turn are delivered more rapidly than those taken orally), its receptor affinity, its rate of dissociation from the receptors and its plasma half-life. Therefore, short-acting drugs that can be inhaled are the most addictive. The harm associated with substance use is often caused by the compulsion associated with high-abuse-liability drugs: the lack of the drug leads to drug-seeking behaviour at the expense of other normal behaviours.

ENVIRONMENTAL FACTORS

The social determinants of health are inversely correlated with substance use disorders. Those who have a lower level of education, who are underemployed and who live in poverty or in impoverished neighbourhoods are at higher risk of developing drug problems. Moreover, depending on the individual's age at the onset of substance use, this use may not only result from, but may also directly affect, the educational level reached and the employment and financial resources available to that individual. Social factors—such as societal and family norms, level of social support and laws that affect the availability of drugs—also have an impact on the development of substance use disorders.

TABLE 1-2

DSM-IV criteria for substance use and substance dependence

CRITERIA FOR SUBSTANCE ABUSE

A. A maladaptive pattern of substance use leading to clinically significant impairment or distress, as manifested by one (or more) of the following, occurring within a 12-month period:

1. recurrent substance use resulting in a failure to fulfill major role obligations at work, school, or home (e.g., repeated absences or poor work performance related to substance use; substance-related absences, suspensions, or expulsions from school; neglect of children or household)
2. recurrent substance use in situations in which it is physically hazardous (e.g., driving an automobile or operating a machine when impaired by substance use.
3. recurrent substance-related legal problems (e.g., arrests for substance-related disorderly conduct)
4. continued substance use despite having persistent or recurrent social or interpersonal problems caused or exacerbated by the effects of the substance (e.g., arguments with a spouse about the consequences of intoxication, physical fights).

B. The symptoms have never met the criteria for substance dependence for this class of substance.

CRITERIA FOR SUBSTANCE DEPENDENCE

A maladaptive pattern of substance use, leading to clinically significant impairment or distress, as manifested by three (or more) of the following, occurring at any time in the same 12-month period:

1. The patient develops tolerance, as defined by either of the following:
   a. a need for markedly increased amounts of the substance to achieve intoxication or the desired effect
   b. markedly diminished effect with continued use of the same amount of the substance.
2. The patient experiences withdrawal, as manifested by either of the following:
   a. the characteristic withdrawal syndrome for the substance
   b. the same (or a closely related) substance being taken to relieve or avoid withdrawal symptoms.
3. The substance is often taken in larger amounts or over a longer period than was intended.
4. There is a persistent desire or unsuccessful efforts to cut down or control substance use.
5. A great deal of time is spent in activities necessary to obtain the substance (e.g., visiting multiple doctors or driving long distances), use the substance (e.g., chain-smoking), or recover from its effects.
6. Important social, occupational, or recreational activities are given up or reduced because of the substance use.
7. The substance use is continued despite knowledge of having a persistent or recurrent physical or psychological problem that is likely to have been caused or exacerbated by the substance (e.g., current cocaine use despite recognition of cocaine-induced depression, or continued drinking despite recognition that an ulcer was made worse by alcohol consumption).

The vector of this disease is the supplier, such as a pusher of street drugs. A supplier's actions not only affect a host (by pressuring a vulnerable person to use a drug) but can also affect the purity of the drug (e.g., cutting heroin with white powders, such as baking soda, to increase the total street price of a given quantity) and the environment that makes drug use possible (e.g., shooting galleries, involvement with organized crime). In the case of legal drugs such as tobacco and alcohol, the manufacturers serve as the vector; their tactics to increase drug use can have similar effects. For example, tobacco manufacturers make so-called "mild" cigarettes that lead people who smoke to take deeper breaths in order to get the same level of nicotine—thereby increasing the harm from smoking. They also manipulate the environment by opposing bylaws restricting smoking (which have been shown to benefit both people who smoke and those who do not), thereby creating a market in which young people can more easily get addicted.

Overview of addiction treatment

TREATMENT FACTORS

Addiction treatment fundamentally addresses the disease continuum. Although most people who use drugs do not develop dependence, a minority do develop substantial problems. Most do not seek treatment and may recover spontaneously but, untreated, the disease can be fatal and/or associated with excess morbidity. Recovery is best viewed as a non-linear process that includes relapse as a normal part of the process.

The treatment of Type 2 diabetes mellitus is a useful analogy for physicians in their approach to treating addictions. Like substance dependence, diabetes is caused by a combination of host, agent and environmental factors (McLellan et al., 2000). The first step in treatment involves a behavioural or psychosocial intervention of diet and exercise. If this intervention fails to adequately modify blood sugars, the next step involves the introduction of pharmacotherapy. In some severe cases, especially those with complications (such as premature coronary disease), pharmacotherapy is commenced at the same time as the behavioural intervention. The goal is not to cure the person of diabetes but to mitigate the harm associated with the disease by maintaining blood sugars within a narrow range. The focus is on titrating interventions, both behavioural as well as pharmacological (e.g., referral to a specialist, addition of insulin, monitoring outcome and preventing complications). Similarly, addiction treatment requires an interdisciplinary group of various health care practitioners working together to help the patient achieve his or her treatment goal.

As with other medical conditions, the development of a positive doctor-patient relationship is the basis of successful treatment. Therefore, it is important for physicians to be non-judgmental and patient-centred in their approach and to use counselling methods that empower patients to develop a healthy therapeutic relationship with their care providers. This attitude is especially important for drug treatment because of the stigma so often experienced by patients, even when they are seeking help.

Treatment can be understood along three main dimensions:

- modality (e.g., pharmacotherapy, mutual aid, self-help, inpatient/outpatient behavioural therapies, agonist maintenance therapies)
- intensity (e.g., brief, short-term, long-term)
- situation in the disease time course (e.g., early, late).

The goal of treatment is to induce a remission and then, wherever possible, maintain it in a complete, sustained way.

There are two key philosophies that guide treatment. The more traditional philosophy, known as abstinence-based treatment, typically involves intolerance of any use of drugs, often with little patient choice, and takes a confrontational, even punitive, approach to ongoing drug use. But the newer philosophy of harm reduction, which first evolved in response to the HIV epidemic, has been gaining ground.

Harm reduction is defined as "any program or policy designed to reduce drug-related harm without requiring the cessation of drug use. Interventions may be targeted at the individual, the family, community or society" (CAMH, 2002). This approach involves engaging the patient in the process, using a patient-centred approach, and focusing on improvement in all domains of a patient's life, even though there may be ongoing drug use.

Agonist-based therapies such as methadone maintenance are considered to be harm reduction interventions because the patient is still dependent on opioids. However, many programs incorporate punitive policies, such as discharge for drug use, rather than pragmatic solutions such as appropriate titration of the dose of methadone, use of contingency management and increased counselling to address other barriers to recovery.

Early treatment for most addictions involves a period of withdrawal management. Depending on the available resources and the medical and social complexity of the case, withdrawal may be accomplished on either an outpatient or inpatient basis. The goal is to overcome withdrawal safely, with or without pharmacotherapy. The withdrawal stage also offers the patient an opportunity to take stock, begin treatment planning and become socially stable with respect to housing, finances, legal issues and so on. Most acute withdrawal remits within 10 days if the patient tolerates the process (see the section "Withdrawal from opioids" on page 14 in Chapter 2). Acute withdrawal is most often followed by intense cravings for drug use, which are associated with relapse unless other strategies are used to maintain abstinence.

At this point, patients should ideally enter an intensive or post-acute phase of treatment in which they gain a better understanding of their substance use triggers and develop skills to maintain a drug-free life. This phase usually lasts 21 days and is followed by an indefinite period of aftercare. Longer programs—therapeutic communities lasting three to 12 months—benefit a select few who are willing to invest the time and live away from their families and jobs.

For many heroin-dependent individuals, despite many cycles of withdrawal and treatment, the disease remains active or even increases in severity. Treatment with agonists such as methadone has become the standard of care for such patients.

TREATMENT MODALITIES

There are two main treatment modalities: pharmacotherapy and psychosocial interventions. Integrating both approaches leads to superior outcomes for most addictive disorders.

Pharmacotherapy

Several classes of medication are used to treat addiction:

- In *agonist substitution therapy*, a safer and longer-acting drug of the same class is substituted for the addicting drug (e.g., methadone for opioids or the nicotine patch for tobacco).
- *Anti-craving medication* acts on neurotransmitters to reduce the reinforcing properties of the drug (e.g., naltrexone for alcohol) or relieve subacute withdrawal symptoms (e.g., bupropion).
- *Antagonist therapy* blocks the action of the drug of abuse (e.g., naltrexone for opioids).
- *Aversive therapy* causes unpleasant side-effects if the drug is taken (e.g., disulfiram).
- *Psychotropic medications* alter the underlying cognitive and mood states that contribute to substance use in some patients with concurrent disorders (e.g., antidepressants and mood stabilizers).

Psychosocial treatment

The success rates and cost-effectiveness of formal treatment for substance dependence compare favourably with those of treatments for other chronic illnesses; for example, a review of controlled trials found a six-month success rate of 50 per cent (defined as a reduction of more than 50 per cent in the Addiction Severity Index) (O'Brien & McLellan, 1996). Prognosis is better in patients who have a shorter history of substance use, a network of social supports and no concurrent psychiatric illnesses or other addictions. Cognitive therapy, therapist-facilitated mutual support groups and motivational interviewing are all effective approaches, and most programs use a combination of all three (Project MATCH Research Group, 1998).

Outpatient programs are effective for socially stable patients with less severe psychosocial or substance use problems. Inpatient treatment is indicated for patients who have been unsuccessful with outpatient treatment, require medical management of withdrawal or live in an unsupportive home environment. Most inpatient programs provide regular follow-up group sessions for up to two years.

Mutual aid groups such as Alcoholics Anonymous (AA) and Narcotics Anonymous (NA) are based on the "12 steps," a set of principles that emphasize personal responsibility and honesty. There are both open AA meetings (which the general public can attend) and closed ones (which only group members attend). Each group member is encouraged to choose a more senior group member as a sponsor.

Membership in AA has many advantages. The meetings are free and easily accessible, and membership can be lifelong—making AA important for relapse prevention. Sponsors and experienced members provide practical advice and support, sometimes making themselves available on evenings and weekends. A close bond frequently develops among group members.

Summary

Addiction is a chronic, relapsing brain disease caused by the complex interplay of host, environment, drug and vector, and it is treatable by interdisciplinary teams. Treatment involves various modalities and different intensities that need to be matched to the time course of the disease, with the goal of inducing and maintaining a remission wherever possible. Recovery is a non-linear process that is facilitated tremendously by the development of a healthy doctor-patient relationship. Comparing addiction treatment to that of other chronic diseases helps to de-stigmatize patients and helps health care practitioners, as well as patients and their families, to understand the goals of treatment and care.

References

American Psychiatric Association (APA). (2004). *Diagnostic and Statistical Manual of Mental Disorders* (4th ed., text revision). Washington, DC: Author.

American Society of Addiction Medicine (ASAM). (2003). *Principles of Addiction Medicine* (3rd ed.). Chevy Chase, MD: Author.

Centre for Addiction and Mental Health (CAMH). (2002). CAMH position on harm reduction: Its meaning and application for substance use issues [web page]. Retrieved from www.camh.net/Public_policy/Public_policy_papers/publicpolicy_harmreduc2002.html.

Hyman, S.E., Malenka, R.C. & Nestler, E.J. (2006). Neural mechanisms of addiction: The role of reward-related learning and memory. *Annual Review of Neuroscience, 29*, 565–598.

Hyman, S.E. & Malenka, R.C. (2001). Addiction and the brain: The neurobiology of compulsion and its persistence. *Nature Reviews Neuroscience, 2*, 695–703.

Hyman, S.E. (2005). Addiction: A disease of learning and memory. *American Journal of Psychiatry, 162*, 1414–1422.

Kalivas, P.W. & Volkow, N.D. (2005). The neural basis of addiction: A pathology of motivation and choice. *American Journal of Psychiatry, 162*, 1403–1413.

Lachman, H.M. (2006). An overview of the genetics of substance use disorders. *Current Psychiatry Reports, 8*, 133–143.

McLellan, A.T., Lewis, D.C., O'Brien, C.P. & Kleber, H.D. (2000). Drug dependence, a chronic medical illness: Implications for treatment, insurance, and outcomes evaluation. *Journal of the American Medical Association, 284*, 1689–1695.

O'Brien, C.P. & McLellan, A.T. (1996). Myths about the treatment of addiction. *The Lancet, 347*, 237–240.

Project MATCH Research Group. (1998). Matching alcoholism treatments to client heterogeneity: Project MATCH three-year drinking outcomes. *Alcoholism: Clinical and Experimental Research, 22*, 1300–1311.

Volkow, N.D. (2005). What do we know about drug addiction? *American Journal of Psychiatry, 162*, 1401–1402.

Volkow, N.D. & Li, T.K. (2005). Drugs and alcohol: Treating and preventing abuse, addiction and their medical consequences. *Pharmacology and Therapeutics, 108*, 3–17.

CHAPTER 2

Opioid dependence

This chapter describes various aspects of opioid dependence. It begins by explaining the diagnostic criteria, as well as the pharmacology of and risks associated with opioid use. It also covers the diagnostic criteria and symptoms of opioid withdrawal. The chapter concludes with an overview of the treatment options for opioid withdrawal.

DSM-IV criteria for opioid dependence

According to the widely agreed upon diagnostic criteria for substance dependence in the DSM-IV (see Table 1-2) a person considered to be dependent on opioids may or may not display evidence of physical dependence in the form of tolerance or withdrawal, but must be experiencing significant physical, psychological or social sequelae from opioid use that interfere significantly in his or her life.

There is a small population of opioid users who do not use daily or are not physically dependent even though they inject opioids. Moreover, some patients use only oral prescription opioids (Brands et al., 2002).

Oral prescription users may obtain prescriptions from multiple doctors or from drug dealers, take large doses and exhibit signs of physical dependence; however, they may not experience the same physical, psychological and social sequelae as injection heroin users. Therefore, regardless of type of opioid or route of administration, physicians are expected to consider the full spectrum of drug use and ensure that the patient entering methadone maintenance treatment (MMT) meets the criteria for opioid dependence, presented in Table 2-1.

TABLE 2-1

DSM-IV diagnostic criteria for opioid dependence

The DSM-IV specifies that three or more of the following symptoms must occur at some time during a 12-month period and cause significant impairment or distress in order to meet the diagnostic criteria for opioid dependence:

Tolerance—The individual either has to use increasingly higher amounts of the drug over time in order to achieve the same drug effect or finds that the same amount of the drug has much less of an effect over time than before.

Withdrawal—The individual either experiences a characteristic abstinence syndrome (i.e., opioid-specific withdrawal) or uses opioids or similar-acting drugs in order to avoid or relieve withdrawal symptoms.

Loss of control—The individual either repeatedly uses more opioids than planned or uses the opioids over longer periods of time than planned.

Inability to stop using—The individual has either unsuccessfully attempted to cut down or stop using the opioids or has a persistent desire to stop using.

Time—The individual spends a lot of time obtaining opioids, getting money to buy opioids, using opioids, being under the influence of opioids and recovering from the effects of opioids.

Interference with activities—The individual either gives up or reduces the amount of time involved in recreational activities, social activities and/or occupational activities.

Harm to self—The individual continues to use opioids despite having a physical or psychological problem (e.g., depression) that is caused or made worse by the opioid use.

Adapted from the *Diagnostic and Statistical Manual of Mental Disorders*, Fourth Edition, Text Revision (Copyright 2000). American Psychiatric Association.

DIFFERENTIAL DIAGNOSIS OF OPIOID DEPENDENCE

It can be extremely difficult to diagnose opioid dependence in the context of a poorly treated chronic pain problem. These patients can meet the criteria without necessarily being addicted or requiring addiction treatment (see the section "Chronic pain" on page 109 in Chapter 12). At best, the diagnosis is made prospectively, with the physician optimizing the medications, setting appropriate boundaries and observing the patient's response. Factors that may alert the physician to an addiction are dependence on other non-opioids (such as cocaine or other stimulants), alcohol dependence and use of illicit opioids (such as heroin).

Prevalence and consequences of opioid dependence

General-population surveys find a prevalence of opioid dependence of less than one per cent. However, these surveys tend to miss people who are homeless or who do not have telephones.

The consequences of opioid dependence include not only direct health effects—such as the development of HIV or infective endocarditis due to the route of administration, overdose and respiratory arrest—but also social consequences, such as criminality. There are also associated consequences, such as family breakdown, loss or lack of employment and other health effects. The cost associated with an untreated heroin-dependent patient is calculated to be over $44,000 annually—the annual social cost generated by 114 daily opioid users not currently in or seeking treatment for their addiction is calculated at over $5.086 million, mostly due to crime victimization (44.6 per cent) and law enforcement (42.4 per cent), followed by productivity losses (seven per cent) and the use of health care (6.1 per cent) (Wall et al., 2000). Therefore, this is a public health problem that requires a pragmatic approach to treatment.

Pharmacology of opioids

OPIATES

Opioids are a pharmacological class of drugs that have morphine-like activity and bind to opioid receptors in the body. The naturally occurring compounds derived from opium are known as opiates. These include morphine and codeine, which were isolated and purified in 1806 and 1832 respectively. Opium's abilities to relieve pain, cause drowsiness, relieve diarrhea and induce a pleasant dreamy state have been known and used for over 4,000 years.

SEMI-SYNTHETICS AND SYNTHETICS

The isolation and purification of opiates led to the development of semi-synthetic and synthetic substances with morphine-like effects, which were developed in the course of efforts to find substances that could relieve pain without inducing withdrawal when discontinued. Semi-synthetic opioids include heroin (diacetylmorphine); synthetic opioids include oxycodone, meperidine, buprenorphine and methadone. Also included in this group are endogenous opioids, substances with morphine-like effects that are found in our bodies. These include the endorphins (the term is a contraction of "endogenous" and "morphine"), enkephalins and dynorphin.

The earliest semi-synthetics included diacetylmorphine, which was developed by Bayer in 1898 and given the brand name Heroin, and hydromorphone, developed in the early 1900s and now most commonly known by the brand name Dilaudid.

Among the earliest synthetics are meperidine and methadone (originally named Hoechst 10820), which were developed in Germany by IG Farbenindustrie in 1939 and 1941 respectively. After German patents were requisitioned by the allies following World War II, the formula for methadone was exploited by many companies, including Eli Lilly in the United States, which marketed it as a pain reliever under the brand name Dolophine (from the Latin word for pain, *dolor*).

In addition to those opioids already mentioned, the opioid group of medications also includes hydrocodone, diphenoxylate and dextromethorphan. Opioids are included in a variety of over-the-counter and prescribed medications widely available from pharmacies, including the following:

- MS Contin (contains morphine)
- Tylenol 1 to 4 (contains codeine)
- Dilaudid (contains hydromorphone)
- Demerol (contains meperidine)
- Tussionex (contains hydrocodone)
- Percodan (contains oxycodone)
- Lomotil (contains diphenoxylate)
- Benylin DM (contains dextromethorphan).

In Canada, medications containing diacetylmorphine (i.e., heroin) are illegal.

OPIOID ANTAGONISTS AND AGONIST/ ANTAGONISTS

As their name suggests, opioid antagonists are substances that interact with opioid receptors to block the action of opioid drugs, preventing an opioid from producing its usual effect. Some antagonists, such as naloxone, are useful in the emergency treatment of individuals who have taken a potentially lethal overdose of an opioid. Another antagonist, naltrexone, has been used to "protect" individuals who were formerly physically dependent on opioids but are now drug-free. While they are taking naltrexone, these individuals will not experience opioid effects if they use an opioid.

Some drugs, such as pentazocine and buprenorphine, have both opioid agonist and antagonist properties—that is, they have a combination of morphine-like and morphine-antagonizing properties. Such drugs are thought to react at the site of more than one type of receptor, exerting a different effect through each.

MECHANISM OF ACTION OF OPIOIDS

Opioids act by binding to endogenous opioid receptors in the peripheral and central nervous systems. Therefore they are used as analgesics, antitussives and acute anti-dyspneics for pulmonary edema. The psychoactive effects of opioids range from mild mood levelling to profound euphoria and a sense of inner peace. Autonomic effects include miosis, sweating, decreased gastrointestinal motility, constipation and urinary retention. The analgesic and psychoactive duration of action for heroin and most prescription opioids ranges from three to six hours. Sustained-release preparations (e.g., MS Contin and Kadian) induce analgesia for eight to 24 hours.

In general, the side-effects of opioids (e.g., drowsiness and constipation) are due to their actions in the nervous system. The side-effects are often acute, and many patients develop tolerance to the effects of opioids.

TOLERANCE

As described in Chapter 1, tolerance is the need for higher doses of a drug in order to achieve the same effect, or the reduction of the effect with use of the same dose over time. It is caused by changes in the number and sensitivity of receptors—changes that allow the body to compensate for a drug's effect. This phenomenon occurs in all organ systems of the body. Opioid tolerance is of particular relevance in relation to certain effects, as described below.

Analgesic effects

Tolerance to the analgesic effects of opioids develops very slowly, and patients taking opioid analgesics for chronic non-malignant pain are often able to remain on the same dose for months or even years. Therefore, patients who require frequent dose increases for uncontrolled pain may have opioid-non-responsive pain, they may be suffering from an underlying untreated pathology and/or they may have developed a substance dependence disorder.

Psychoactive effects

Tolerance to the psychoactive effects of opioids develops quickly. This phenomenon, coupled with the short half-lives of most opioids, makes them prone to abuse. People who are seeking the mood-altering effects of opioids are driven to rapidly escalate their doses until they reach a daily amount that satisfies them—this amount varies from individual to individual.

Gastrointestinal and respiratory effects

Patients rarely develop significant tolerance to the effects of opioids on gastrointestinal motility. Substantial but incomplete tolerance to the respiratory-depressant effects of opioids develops over time. This makes opioid overdose particularly dangerous, especially in those with an already compromised respiratory drive due either to illness (e.g., chronic obstructive pulmonary disease [COPD]) or concurrent use of drugs from a different class with respiratory-depressant effects (e.g., benzodiazepines, alcohol, barbiturates).

Risks of opioid use

OVERDOSE

Risk factors for overdose

- A number of factors have been shown to contribute to the risk of overdose, including:
- dose and potency of the opioid
- parenteral administration
- lack of tolerance to opioids (note that tolerance can decline significantly within three days of last use)
- timing of administration (risk increases if opioid is taken shortly before onset of sleep)
- setting of administration (risk increases if opioid is taken in unfamiliar surroundings)
- lack of pain
- use of other sedative or psychoactive drug
- altered metabolism due to drug use or to renal or hepatic impairment
- age (risk is higher in the elderly)
- cardiorespiratory illness.

Symptoms of overdose

Opioid overdose is characterized by decreased levels of consciousness, decreased respiratory rate, bradycardia and miosis. Sedation is the first sign of an overdose. The patient has pinpoint pupils, may be sweating and appears to be drowsy and "nodding off" (i.e., momentarily falling asleep), with slurred, drawling speech, ataxia and sometimes emotional lability. Later signs include coma, shallow breathing with a respiratory rate of less than 12 breaths per minute, bradycardia and cyanosis. Long-acting opioids, particularly methadone, can have a gradual, insidious onset of symptoms. Overdose is sometimes complicated by non-cardiogenic pulmonary edema.

Withdrawal from opioids

The phenomenon of tolerance to a drug is physiological and leads to physical dependence on the drug. When the drug is suddenly stopped, the physiological adaptations do not disappear immediately. In the drug's absence, they appear as withdrawal symptoms and signs, which are generally the opposite of the drug's direct effects. Withdrawal symptoms can appear within a few hours to several days after discontinuation, depending primarily on the drug's elimination half-life. Note that if a person experiences withdrawal, it does not necessarily mean that the person has a diagnosis of opioid dependence as defined in the DSM-IV.

Withdrawal occurs not only with drugs of abuse but with any drug that can induce physiological tolerance (e.g., beta blockers, steroids such as cortisone, and many antidepressants, especially SSRIs [selective serotonin reuptake inhibitors]). Sudden withdrawal from some drugs of abuse can be harmful or even fatal. Opioid withdrawal in adults is relatively safe; however, opioid withdrawal in neonates can be fatal.

All drugs of abuse, including opioids, release dopamine in the nucleus accumbens when they are taken acutely. This is thought to be the final common pathway for the experience of euphoria. With repeated administration over time, individuals develop tolerance to the euphorigenic effects, and they may attempt to increase the dose or try to reset their tolerance levels by not taking the drug for a short while. When levels of the drug in the brain fall, patients become dysphoric (the opposite of euphoric) and anxious, and they crave the drug.

People who ingest, inject or inhale opioid agonists on a regular basis quickly develop signs of physical dependence, including tolerance and withdrawal. Over time, many individuals who are opioid dependent will continue to use drugs to relieve the discomfort of withdrawal more than for any associated euphoria.

DIAGNOSIS OF OPIOID WITHDRAWAL

The clinical criteria for the diagnosis of opioid withdrawal as described in the DSM-IV are presented in Table 2-2.

TABLE 2-2

DSM-IV criteria for opioid withdrawal

A. Either of the following:

1. cessation of (or reduction in) opioid use that has been heavy and prolonged (several weeks or longer)
2. administration of an opioid antagonist after a period of opioid use.

B. Three (or more) of the following develop within minutes to several days after Criterion A:

1. dysphoric mood
2. nausea or vomiting
3. muscle aches
4. lacrimation or rhinorrhea
5. pupillary dilation, piloerection or sweating
6. diarrhea
7. yawning
8. fever
9. insomnia.

C. The symptoms in Criterion B cause clinically significant distress or impairment in social, occupational or other important areas of functioning.

D. The symptoms are not due to a general medical condition and are not better accounted for by another mental disorder.

TIME COURSE OF WITHDRAWAL

The time course of opioid withdrawal is related to the elimination half-life of the agonist being used by the patient. For agents with a short half-life, such as heroin, morphine, codeine or oxycodone, withdrawal begins within hours of the cessation or reduction in use of the drug.

The symptoms of withdrawal peak in intensity within two to three days after the last use and largely resolve within five days; however, some people are symptomatic for up to 10 days after the last use. People with long-term psychological dependence on opioids may experience insomnia and dysphoria for months afterwards (Kanof et al., 1993), perhaps because of suppression of endogenous ligands (i.e., endorphins) or a structural derangement of the opioid receptor system (Dole, 1988; Kreek, 1987).

SIGNS AND SYMPTOMS OF WITHDRAWAL

Physical symptoms

Opioid withdrawal is characterized by flu-like symptoms, the most distinct of which are myalgias. The myalgias are described as diffuse muscle aches, cramps and an electric or "creepy-crawly" feeling. Other physical symptoms include nausea, abdominal cramps and chills.

Objective signs

Objective signs are generally not seen except on day two or three after abrupt withdrawal from large doses of opioids. The most common sign is restlessness: the patient is uncomfortable and may be huddled over and rocking or unable to sit quietly. Other signs include:

- lacrimation
- rhinorrhea and dilated pupils
- abdominal tenderness
- vomiting
- diarrhea
- tachycardia and hypertension (mild)
- sweating
- yawning
- chills and piloerection (elicited by running a fingernail down the patient's arm).

Psychological symptoms

Psychological symptoms of opioid withdrawal include:

- insomnia (often severe and prolonged)
- fatigue
- anxiety and depression
- drug craving.

Opioid withdrawal is frightening and unpleasant. Patients frequently cite withdrawal avoidance as their main reason for ongoing opioid use. Withdrawal from methadone, and probably other opioids, is associated with an organic mood syndrome. Depressed mood can occur in some patients at the end of their methadone dosing interval (Dyer et al., 2001).

RISKS OF OPIOID WITHDRAWAL

Unlike sedative withdrawal, opioid withdrawal is not accompanied by serious medical complications, except in pregnant women and neonates. The two major risks of withdrawal in non-pregnant patients are suicide and overdose.

Suicide

Withdrawal-associated dysphoria can lead to suicide, especially in patients who do not have access to opioids to relieve withdrawal symptoms (e.g., prison inmates).

Overdose

Withdrawal is accompanied by a rapid loss of tolerance. Medically managed withdrawal actually increases the risk of overdose through this mechanism (Strang et al., 2003).

It is crucial to have a comprehensive treatment plan in place before undertaking a medically managed withdrawal from methadone, and to warn patients about the risk of overdose if they relapse.

Iatrogenic withdrawal

Withdrawal of especially severe intensity can also be precipitated abruptly by the administration of an opioid antagonist such as naloxone or naltrexone to a patient who is opioid dependent.

OVERVIEW OF WITHDRAWAL MANAGEMENT OPTIONS

Treatment of withdrawal is a necessary first step for people for whom MMT is not appropriate, not desired or not available. Three commonly used therapies for opioid withdrawal in Canada are:

- tapering doses of methadone
- tapering doses of prescription opioids
- clonidine.

Regardless of the treatment protocol, managed withdrawal alone usually does not result in long-term abstinence (Amato et al., 2004).

Furthermore, managed withdrawal significantly increases the risk of overdose on relapse. It should always be combined with enrolment in a drug rehabilitation program. Psychosocial support from friends and families is also extremely important to successful long-term recovery.

For more detail about opioid withdrawal management, see Chapter 6, "Abstinence-based interventions for opioid withdrawal."

References

Amato, L., Davoli, M., Ferri, M., Gowing, L. & Perucci, C.A. (2004). Effectiveness of interventions on opiate withdrawal treatment: An overview of systematic reviews. *Drug and Alcohol Dependence, 73* (3), 219–226.

APA (2004). *Diagnostic and Statistical Manual of Mental Disorders* (4th ed., text revision). Washington, DC: Author.

Brands, B., Blake, J. & Marsh, D. (2002). Changing patient characteristics with increased methadone maintenance availability. *Drug and Alcohol Dependence, 66* (1), 11–20.

Dole, V.P. (1988). Implications of methadone maintenance for theories of narcotic addiction. *Journal of the American Medical Association, 260* (20), 3025–3029.

Dyer, K.R., White, J.M., Foster, D.J., Bochner, F., Menelaou, A. & Somogyi, A.A. (2001). The relationship between mood state and plasma methadone concentration in maintenance patients. *Journal of Clinical Psychopharmacology, 21* (1), 78–84.

Kanof, P.D., Aronson, M.J. & Ness, R. (1993). Organic mood syndrome associated with detoxification from methadone maintenance. *American Journal of Psychiatry, 150* (3), 423–428.

Kreek, M.J. (1987). Tolerance and dependence: Implications for the pharmacological treatment of addiction. *NIDA Research Monograph 76,* 53–62.

Strang, J., McCambridge, J., Best, D., Beswick, T., Bearn, J., Rees, S. et al. (2003). Loss of tolerance and overdose mortality after inpatient opiate detoxification: Follow up study. *British Medical Journal, 326* (7396), 959–960.

Wall, R., Rehm, J., Fischer, B., Brands, B., Gliksman, L., Stewart, J. et al. (2000). Social costs of untreated opioid dependence. *Journal of Urban Health, 77* (4), 688–722.

CHAPTER 3

Effectiveness of methadone maintenance treatment

This chapter describes the benefits and limitations of methadone maintenance treatment (MMT) and explains the various factors that contribute to its success as a treatment for opioid-dependent patients.

Benefits of MMT

Over the past four decades, MMT has been evaluated in numerous randomized trials and large prospective studies involving tens of thousands of patients. The results are strong and consistent: MMT is highly effective in reducing heroin use and its consequences, including incarceration and death from suicide and violence. Methadone, when prescribed as part of a comprehensive rehabilitation program, is effective in decreasing the spread of HIV (Metzger et al., 1993; Des Jarlais et al., 1994), decreasing injection drug use (Ball & Ross, 1991), improving psychosocial functioning, decreasing crime rates and increasing employment rates in treated versus untreated people who are addicted to heroin (Powers & Anglin, 1993).

As described in Chapter 4, methadone has several properties that make it ideally suited as a treatment for opioid dependence—it is potent, has a slow onset and long duration of action, causes cross-tolerance and can be easily distinguished from heroin with urine toxicology.

MMT AND HEROIN USE

When MMT is measured against no treatment, the results are impressive. In an early randomized trial conducted by Dole and Joseph, the control group was 92 times more likely to be using heroin on a daily basis (Dole & Joseph, 1978). A prospective study by Ball and Ross (1991) found that prior to MMT the arrest rate was 200 per 100 person-years (i.e., patients were arrested twice per year on average). After these patients entered MMT, the arrest rate fell to two per 100 person-years.

Few medical treatments have approached the effectiveness of methadone in reducing mortality. A number of prospective studies have demonstrated that the mortality rate of people who use heroin and who are in MMT is three or four times lower than the rate of untreated people who use heroin, due primarily to fewer deaths from overdose and suicide (Gearing & Schweitzer, 1974; Caplehorn et al., 1994; Sanchez-Carbonell & Seus, 2000; Frischer et al., 1997; Scherbaum et al., 2002; Caplehorn et al., 1996). The overall mortality rate of people who use heroin declines sharply with entry into treatment and climbs again with discharge (Bell & Zador, 2000; Zanis & Woody, 1998; Buster et al., 2002).

Physiological improvement in various neuroendocrine systems, such as normalization of FSH/LH secretion and return of normal menstruation (Blinick, 1968), has also been observed among MMT patients.

MMT AND HIV

A systematic review concluded that rates of needle use and needle sharing decline by 50 per cent or more after patients enrol in MMT (Sullivan et al., 2005). As a consequence, MMT dramatically reduces seroconversion rates in areas of rapidly rising HIV incidence. In one 18-month study of people who inject heroin and are seronegative, only three per cent of the MMT cohort seroconverted, compared to 22 per cent of the untreated cohort (Sullivan et al., 2005). MMT also reduces the HIV transmission from injection drug users to the general population. HIV-positive women on methadone have been shown to reduce their number of sexual partners and their needle sharing (Thiede et al., 2000; Wong et al., 2003; Grella et al., 1996).

MMT VS. TAPERING AND NON-PHARMACOLOGICAL TREATMENT

The treatment effects of MMT are strong and robust, even when measured against intensive non-pharmacological treatments. For example, a Cochrane systematic review (Mattick et al., 2003) of six randomized clinical trials found that treatment retention rates were three times higher with MMT than with non-pharmacological treatments, and rates of heroin use were three times lower. In a randomized controlled trial comparing MMT to methadone tapering, the maintenance group had reduced heroin use, HIV risk factors and criminal behaviour, even though the tapering group had intensive counselling (Sees et al., 2000).

MMT AND OTHER DRUG USE

A concern sometimes raised about MMT is that patients will switch their addiction from heroin to some other harmful substance such as cocaine. Even if this does occur on occasion, evidence suggests that, overall, substance use declines substantially for all classes of drugs, except alcohol and nicotine. One large prospective study (Fairbank et al., 1993) found a reduction in the use of cocaine, amphetamines, illegal methadone, sedatives and marijuana after MMT enrolment. The extent of the decline was considerably less than for opioids, probably because methadone has minimal or no direct pharmacological effect on reducing craving or withdrawal symptoms for non-opioid drugs. It is not known why alcohol use does not decline.

Limitations of MMT

While the effectiveness of MMT is remarkable, it is not 100 per cent. In British Columbia from 1996 to 1999, the one-year treatment retention rate was only 52 per cent, although if people who dropped out and later re-entered MMT are included the rate climbs to 76 per cent (Anderson & Warren, 2004). MMT programs need to implement and evaluate strategies to improve retention rates, for example by offering counselling and social services, optimal methadone dosing and flexible clinic policies (Anderson & Warren, 2004; Farre et al., 2002; Goldstein et al., 2002; Amato et al., 2004; Gaughwin et al., 1998).

A further challenge that limits the effectiveness of MMT is availability. It is estimated that only 20 per cent of opioid-dependent patients are on MMT in Canada (Fischer, 2000), and in many regions of Canada MMT is unavailable. To improve program effectiveness, there should be better support for primary care physicians who attempt to provide MMT, through training opportunities, access to clinical expertise and assistance with facilities and personnel.

FACTORS THAT AFFECT MMT

Research has determined that the following factors all have an effect on drug use and treatment retention in MMT:

- counselling
- urine drug screening
- contingency management through daily dispensing and take-home doses
- clinic discharge policies.

(These studies are discussed more fully in later chapters focusing on specific MMT-related topics.) The fact that non-opioid drug use declines with MMT confirms that non-pharmacological factors are also important.

LIMITATIONS OF THE RESEARCH

Virtually all existing MMT research has been conducted on heroin-dependent patients. Yet evidence suggests that the prevalence of prescription opioid dependence is increasing rapidly, and that such dependence is a common reason for admission to MMT in Canada (Brands et al., 2002).

Although there has been little research in this area, the benefit-risk ratio of MMT for prescription opioids may be different than for heroin. For example, it seems possible that people who use prescription opioids are at lower risk for suicide, violence, incarceration and HIV than are people who use heroin. At the same time, the risk of complications from MMT among people who use prescription opioids may be higher if, on average, they have a lower baseline opioid tolerance or are on sedating medications.

There is therefore an even stronger onus on physicians to ensure that prescription opioid users meet DSM-IV criteria for dependence, are more likely to benefit from methadone treatment than other forms of treatment, and are highly tolerant to opioids. Definitive research is also lacking on fundamental policy issues in MMT, such as the frequency of urine drug screens and the optimal schedule of take-home doses. (These issues are discussed in greater detail in later chapters.)

Summary

MMT has been shown to reduce illicit heroin use and its associated morbidity and mortality. The benefits of methadone treatment for prescription opioid users have not been extensively studied. Further efforts are required to improve treatment retention and treatment access in Canada.

References

Amato, L., Minozzi, S., Davoli, M., Vecchi, S., Ferri, M. & Mayet, S. (2004). Psychosocial combined with agonist maintenance treatments versus agonist maintenance treatments alone for treatment of opioid dependence. *Cochrane Database of Systematic Reviews, 4*, CD004147.

Anderson, J.F. & Warren, L.D. (2004). Client retention in the British Columbia Methadone Program, 1996–1999. *Canadian Journal of Public Health, 95* (2), 104–109.

Ball, J.C. & Ross, A. (1991). *The Effectiveness of Methadone Maintenance Treatment: Patients, Programs, Services and Outcomes.* New York: Springer.

Bell, J. & Zador, D. (2000). A risk-benefit analysis of methadone maintenance treatment. *Drug Safety, 22* (3), 179–190.

Blinick, G., (1968). Menstrual function and pregnancy in narcotic addicts treated with methadone. *Nature, 219*, 180.

Brands, B., Blake, J. & Marsh, D. (2002). Changing patient characteristics with increased methadone maintenance availability. *Drug and Alcohol Dependence, 66* (1), 11–20.

Buster, M.C., van Brussel, G.H. & van den Brink, W. (2002). An increase in overdose mortality during the first 2 weeks after entering or re-entering methadone treatment in Amsterdam. *Addiction, 97* (8), 993–1001.

Caplehorn, J.R., Dalton, M.S., Cluff, M.C. & Petrenas, A.M. (1994). Retention in methadone maintenance and heroin addicts' risk of death. *Addiction, 89* (2), 203–209.

Caplehorn, J.R., Dalton, M.S., Haldar, F., Petrenas, A.M. & Nisbet, J.G. (1996). Methadone maintenance and addicts' risk of fatal heroin overdose. *Substance Use and Misuse, 31* (2), 177–196.

Des Jarlais, D.C., Friedman, S.R., Sotheran, J.L., Wenston, J., Marmor, M., Yancovitz, S.R. et al. (1994). Continuity and change within an HIV epidemic: Injecting drug users in New York City, 1984 through 1992. *Journal of the American Medical Association, 271*, 121–127.

Dole, V.P. & Joseph, H. (1978). Long-term outcome of patients treated with methadone maintenance. *Annals of the New York Academy of Sciences, 311*, 181–189.

Fairbank, J.A., Dunteman, G.H. & Condelli, W.S. (1993). Do methadone patients substitute other drugs for heroin? Predicting substance use at 1-year follow-up. *American Journal of Drug and Alcohol Abuse, 19* (4), 465–474.

Farre, M., Mas, A., Torrens, M., Moreno, V. & Cami, J. (2002). Retention rate and illicit opioid use during methadone maintenance interventions: A meta-analysis. *Drug and Alcohol Dependence, 65* (3), 283–290.

Fischer, B. (2000). Prescriptions, power and politics: The turbulent history of methadone maintenance in Canada. *Journal of Public Health Policy, 21* (2), 187–210.

Frischer, M., Goldberg, D., Rahman, M. & Berney, L. (1997). Mortality and survival among a cohort of drug injectors in Glasgow, 1982–1994. *Addiction, 92* (4) 419–427.

Gaughwin, M., Solomon, P. & Ali, R. (1998). Correlates of retention on the South Australian Methadone Program 1981–91. *Australian and New Zealand Journal of Public Health 22* (7), 771–776.

Gearing, F.R. & Schweitzer, M.D. (1974). An epidemiologic evaluation of long-term methadone maintenance treatment for heroin addiction. *American Journal of Epidemiology, 100,* 101–112.

Goldstein, M.F., Deren, S., Kang, S.Y., Des Jarlais, D.C. & Magura, S. (2002). Evaluation of an alternative program for MMTP drop-outs: Impact on treatment re-entry. *Drug and Alcohol Dependence, 66* (2), 181–187.

Grella, C.E., Anglin, D. & Annon, J.J. (1996). HIV risk behaviors among women in methadone maintenance treatment. *Substance Use and Misuse, 31* (3), 277–301.

Mattick, R.P., Breen, C., Kimber, J. & Davoli, M. (2003). Methadone maintenance therapy versus no opioid replacement therapy for opioid dependence. *Cochrane Database of Systematic Reviews, 2,* CD002209.

Metzger, D.S., Woody, G.E., McLellan, A.T., O'Brien C.P., Druley, H. et al. (1993). Human immunodeficiency virus seroconversion among intravenous drug users in- and out-of-treatment: An 18-month prospective follow-up. *Journal of Acquired Immune Deficiency Syndromes, 6* (9), 1049–1056.

Powers, K.I. & Anglin, M.D. (1993). Cumulative versus stabilizing effects of methadone maintenance. *Evaluation Review, 17* (3), 243–270.

Sanchez-Carbonell, X. & Seus, L. (2000). Ten-year survival analysis of a cohort of heroin addicts in Catalonia: The EMETYST project. *Addiction, 95* (6), 941–948.

Scherbaum, N., Specka, M., Hauptmann, G. & Gastpar, M. (2002). Does maintenance treatment reduce the mortality rate of opioid addicts? *Fortschritte der Neurologie-Psychiatrie, 70* (9), 455–461.

Sees, K.L., Delucchi, K.L., Masson, C., Rosen, A., Clark, H.W., Robillard, H. et al. (2000). Methadone maintenance vs 180-day psychosocially enriched detoxification for treatment of opioid dependence: A randomized controlled trial. *Journal of the American Medical Association, 283* (10), 1303–1310.

Sullivan, L.E., Metzger, D.S., Fudala, P.J. & Fiellin, D.A. (2005). Decreasing international HIV transmission: The role of expanding access to opioid agonist therapies for injection drug users. *Addiction, 100* (2), 150–158.

Thiede, H., Hagan, H. & Murrill, C.S. (2000). Methadone treatment and HIV and hepatitis B and C risk reduction among injectors in the Seattle area. *Journal of Urban Health, 77* (3), 331–345.

Wong, K.H., Lee, S.S., Lim, W.L. & Low, H.K. (2003). Adherence to methadone is associated with a lower level of HIV-related risk behaviors in drug users. *Journal of Substance Abuse Treatment, 24* (3), 233–239.

Zanis, D.A. & Woody, G.E. (1998). One-year mortality rates following methadone treatment discharge. *Drug and Alcohol Dependence, 52,* 257–260.

CHAPTER 4

Pharmacology of methadone

This chapter provides a full overview of the pharmacology of methadone and the possible adverse effects of methadone on the patient. It includes a detailed description of many known drug interactions and provides brief clinical tips on managing them.

Pharmacology overview

Methadone, a white, bitter-tasting powder, is a synthetic, orally effective mu receptor opioid agonist with analgesic properties similar to those of morphine. In North America, it is available as 50:50 racemic-methadone ("rac-methadone") both for injection and oral use. Only oral use has been approved for the treatment of opioid dependence in Canada.

ABSORPTION AND BIOAVAILABILITY

Although it can be injected, methadone is readily absorbed from the small intestine and is highly protein-bound (87 per cent) to alpha glycoprotein. There is minimal binding to albumin. The R-isoform is the active enantiomer and has its own pharmacokinetic profile distinct from that of the S-isoform (Foster et al., 2000). It has a greater unbound fraction (173 per cent) than the S-enantiomer.

METABOLISM OF METHADONE

In non-tolerant individuals there is a biexponential decline in serum concentration, with a primary half-life of 14 hours and a secondary half-life of 55 hours (Evans et al., 1973). In tolerant individuals the half-life ranges from 13 to 47 hours (average 25 hours). Methadone is metabolized by N-demethylation in the liver, predominantly by the cytochrome P450 3A4 enzyme system, to its main inactive metabolite: EDDP (2-ethylene-1, 5-dimethyl-3,3-diphenylpyrrolidine) (Baselt, 2000). It may also be metabolized to a lesser extent by the CYP1A2, 2B6, 2C8, 2C9, 2C19 and 2D6 enzyme systems (Antoniou & Tseng, 2002; Wang & DeVane, 2003; Begré et al., 2002; Fuller & Sajatovic, 2001). Methadone is also a weak inhibitor of CYP2D6 (Bertz & Granneman, 1997). Very small, clinically insignificant amounts of the active metabolites methadol and normethadol are also produced when methadone is metabolized (Sullivan et al., 1972).

EXCRETION OF METHADONE

Methadone is excreted by glomerular filtration and is reabsorbed. Reabsorption decreases with increasing acidification of urine. Urinary excretion is the major route of elimination for doses exceeding 55 mg/day. Methadone is also found in sweat and hair but these are not significant routes of elimination.

DOSING GUIDELINES

Daily doses of between 80 and 120 mg are most effective in eliminating illicit opioid use, though some patients may require less and some may require more. Methadone is usually dispensed daily, mixed in orange crystals by a pharmacist or nurse who also witnesses its consumption. In rapid metabolizers or pregnant women, the dose may be split into a bid dosing schedule to prevent withdrawal and relapse.

Individuals are initiated on a dose of no more than 15 to 30 mg/day, which is increased gradually until their illicit opioid use is eliminated. Dose increases are made no more frequently than every five half-lives to prevent accumulation and minimize the risk of overdose and intoxication (Srivastava & Kahan, 2006). As patients become more stable, they may be given take-home doses ("carries"), dispensed in unit daily doses mixed with an orange crystal drink in childproof capped bottles. Since addiction is a chronic disease, treatment is usually indefinite; relapse after discontinuation of MMT ranges between 80 per cent and 90 per cent (McLellan, 1983).

METHADONE FOR CHRONIC PAIN

Due to its long half-life, methadone has been used in the treatment of both malignant and non-malignant chronic pain (Fainsinger et al., 1993). Because its analgesic effect usually lasts only four to six hours, repeated doses might be required for adequate analgesia, which may lead to drug accumulation. Therefore, careful titration and monitoring is required to prevent intoxication and overdose (Lugo et al., 2005; Quigley, 2004; Shir et al., 2001).

Adverse effects of methadone

In general, methadone is very safe and there is very little evidence of long-term organ toxicity. Methadone and other opioids are considerably safer as a class than NSAIDs (non-steroidal anti-inflammatory drugs) (Langman, 2001). There are some possible adverse effects to watch for, as outlined below.

GASTROINTESTINAL EFFECTS

Methadone frequently causes constipation. A bowel routine should be suggested at the onset of therapy (Scholz, 2000; Yuan et al., 1998).

SWEATING

As with other opioids, methadone can cause sweating. This effect is exacerbated by heat and by being in social situations. The sweating is unrelated to withdrawal. If severe, it can be treated with anticholinergics, although these increase the risk of constipation and other effects (Al-Adwani & Basu, 2004; Caflisch et al., 2003).

SEXUAL EFFECTS

Methadone has a marked effect on sexual function and interest level. A survey of methadone patients found dose-related decreases in the frequency of sexual behaviours for both men and women (Crowley & Simpson, 1978). A recent study found that most males on methadone treatment have a low serum testosterone level (Hallinan et al., 2007). Opioids reduce testosterone levels by inhibiting both hypothalamic gonadotrophin-releasing hormone production and testicular testosterone synthesis (Daniell, 2002). Methadone also has variable effects on prolactin, TSH and LH. There is a dose-response relationship between the dose of methadone and orgasmic dysfunction in males (Brown et al., 2005).

All patients on methadone treatment should be asked about sexual dysfunction. Treatment consists of parenteral testosterone (if serum levels are low) or a phosphodiesterase inhibitor. Treatment of the sexual side-effects needs to be guided by the type and severity of the dysfunction. Dose reductions may improve sexual function, but this course of action must be balanced against the risk of withdrawal and relapse. Testosterone supplementation should be reserved for specific cases where the levels are low.

PAIN INTOLERANCE

Patients on chronic opioid therapy may have hypersensitivity to pain (hyperalgesia) (Doverty, White et al., 2001; Pud et al., 2006) and may be more resistant to pain medications. This means that patients on methadone may require higher doses of pain medication for the management of acute pain (Doverty, Somogyi et al., 2001).

COGNITIVE EFFECTS

Methadone patients should be advised to limit their driving or use of machinery during initial titration, after a dose increase, when using other drugs (including alcohol) or if taking other sedating medications. In a standardized driving test, methadone-maintained patients had a longer reaction time and mean decision time than those in the control group; however, there were no significant differences in 20 of the 22 standard tests (Schindler et al., 2004).

Patients on methadone maintenance have shown evidence of cognitive impairment on tests of memory, psychomotor speed and processing information (Darke et al., 2000; Lyvers & Yakimoff, 2003; Mintzer & Stitzer, 2002). The clinical significance of these studies is uncertain as they did not measure cognition during daily performance, nor did they control for other confounding factors such as alcohol dependence, previous head injury or the cognitive effect of repeated overdoses.

Evidence suggests that opioids cause less cognitive impairment than benzodiazepines. In one study, a single dose of morphine (15 mg) caused substantially less impairment of memory and attention than a single dose of lorazepam (1 mg) (O'Neill et al., 2000). In studies with stable cancer patients on opioids, cognitive impairment was subtle, primarily occurring during the initial titration and dose titration periods (Lawlor, 2002).

WEIGHT GAIN

Patients commonly experience weight gain when starting methadone treatment. It appears that methadone may stimulate the intake of food, especially refined sugars (Atkinson, 1987; Bogucka-Bonikowska et al., 2002; Kolarzyk, Chrostek Maj et al., 2005; Kolarzyk, Jenner et al., 2005; Kolarzyk, Pach et al., 2005; Nolan & Scagnelli, 2007). However, the weight gain may also be due to increased caloric intake resulting from decreased drug use, improved mood and improved finances. To prevent obesity, patients starting methadone treatment should receive counselling about exercise, diet and other lifestyle issues.

RESPIRATORY DEPRESSION

The toxicity of methadone is primarily due to its effects on respiration and, to a lesser extent, on its cardiac effects. Patients do not develop complete tolerance to the respiratory-depressant effects of methadone and are therefore prone to dose-dependent respiratory arrest. Mortality depends on the dose of methadone consumed and the individual's level of tolerance. Among non-tolerant individuals, deaths have been associated with doses as low as 50 mg for adults (Dalton & Duncan, 1979; Garriott et al., 1973) and 10 mg for children (Harding-Pink, 1993). In children between the ages of two and six, coma can occur within 90 minutes to three hours and can progress rapidly to respiratory failure and death (Dole et al., 1973).

CARDIAC ARREST/ARRHYTHMIAS

Sudden death in patients on methadone may be related to the development of fatal arrhythmias induced by the methadone (Stimmel, 2003).

QT prolongation

As with other synthetic opioids, there is a dose response relationship between methadone and prolongation of the QT interval. Prolongation of the QTc (corrected QT interval for rate) beyond 500 ms is associated with torsades de pointes, a potentially fatal arrhythmia (Krantz et al., 2002). The QTc may be prolonged due to congenital and acquired structural heart disease, but it is more commonly prolonged by several common medications, including fluoroquinolone and macrolide antibiotics, imidazole antifungal agents, antimalarial agents, phenothiazines, tricyclic antidepressants, antihistamines and other anti-arrhythmic medications. Electrolyte abnormalities, especially hypokalemia, are also commonly associated with the development of torsades de pointes (Krantz & Mehler, 2003).

In one study, the QTc interval did not increase by more than 40 ms in patients on methadone. The mean follow-up QTc interval (±SD) observed in this study (428 ± 21 ms) was well below the 500 ms threshold considered a definite risk for torsades de pointes (Martell et al., 2003). In another study by the same group of investigators, the prolongation was not significant (Krantz et al., 2005). If the increase in QTc crosses this generally accepted threshold (500 ms) it should prompt clinical concern and the contemplation of a dose reduction.

Overall, opioids are essential medications despite the risk of addiction. The World Health Organization has listed methadone as one of the essential drugs to treat opioid dependence (WHO, 2004). If it is prescribed appropriately with an understanding of the risks and benefits, patients can be managed on stable doses of methadone with minimal side-effects.

Drug interactions with methadone

Patients in MMT are often prescribed other medications. In most cases they do not interfere with the methadone treatment; however, patients should be carefully monitored when starting or discontinuing a medication that may interact with methadone. Except for medications that are contraindicated, most interactions can be managed by monitoring for symptoms and making dose adjustments when necessary.

PHARMACODYNAMIC INTERACTIONS

Additive effects

When methadone is combined with a drug with a similar pharmacological profile, the effects may be additive (e.g., potentiation of CNS-depressant effects, constipation, nausea or urinary retention).

The CNS-depressant effects of alcohol and benzodiazepines are additive to those of methadone. Therefore, when methadone and benzodiazepines are taken concurrently, patients are at increased risk for respiratory depression and sedation. This drug interaction has resulted in fatal drug overdose.

Tolerance to some opioid effects, such as respiratory depression, develops very slowly and only partially. Consequently, the additive effects of high doses of methadone and another CNS depressant may have serious consequences. Physicians should take particular care to watch for this interaction at the beginning of methadone treatment and each time the dose is adjusted. As tolerance to the sedative effects of methadone develops, the interaction may become less pronounced.

Another example of an additive effect concerns anticholinergic medications. When given concurrently with methadone, anticholinergics can potentiate the effects on the bowel, causing increased risk of severe constipation, possibly leading to paralytic ileus. This combination can also increase the risk of urinary retention.

Antagonists

A mixed agonist/antagonist, a partial agonist or a pure antagonist will precipitate opioid withdrawal when administered to a patient on MMT. Therefore, these drugs are contraindicated for stable methadone-maintained patients. (For a list, see "Research findings and clinical tips for specific interactions" on page 27.)

However, note that for an overdose of an opioid—including methadone—an antagonist such as naloxone may be life-saving. (See Chapter 2 for more on the pharmacology of opioids.)

PHARMACOKINETIC INTERACTIONS

The effects of induction of methadone metabolism occur slowly as new enzymes are synthesized. The greatest effects generally occur one to two weeks after treatment begins and can result in methadone withdrawal symptoms. In contrast, inhibition of methadone metabolism occurs rapidly, and the effects of toxicity, such as sedation or respiratory distress, can present in as little as one to two days. Patients need to be monitored for a longer period of time to see the effects of induction.

There are few systematic studies of drug interactions with methadone in the literature—much of the information is from clinical case reports. When predicting methadone interactions, physicians and pharmacists need to be aware of the following shortcomings associated with using general cytochrome P450 tables (Moolchan et al., 2001; Davis & Walsh, 2001; Bertz & Granneman, 1997):

- Interactions have been theorized on the basis of liver enzyme alteration. Some of the predicted interactions have been observed clinically, while others have not. For example, ritonavir was predicted to increase methadone effects, but case reports have shown that the opposite occurs.
- Some studies have shown a lack of correlation between changes in methadone plasma levels and the resulting symptoms. For example, MMT patients on efavirenz, which decreases methadone levels, required dose increases, yet MMT patients on nelfinavir, which significantly decreases methadone AUC (the area under the concentration-time curve), did not.
- The magnitude of change in methadone levels seen in studies does not appear to require a corresponding magnitude of dose change. In one study efavirenz decreased methadone AUC by 60 per cent, yet methadone doses were increased by only 22 per cent.

- There is much inter-individual variability in CYP450 metabolism, making predictions based on in vitro information often unreliable.
- Differences in genetic phenotype (e.g., extensive versus poor metabolizers with regard to CYP2D6) can affect drug interactions.
- Other factors may predominate in some interactions, such as competition for protein-binding sites, drug effects on P-glycoprotein, changes in urinary pH or different effects on methadone enantiomers.

GENERAL CLINICAL RECOMMENDATIONS REGARDING DRUG INTERACTIONS

Clinicians should keep in mind the following general recommendations regarding drug interactions with methadone:

- Carefully consider all medications a patient is taking so that treatment of other medical conditions (e.g., HIV or tuberculosis) is not compromised.
- When methadone dose increases are necessary, make adjustments slowly and in small increments to avoid cumulative toxicity.
- With pharmacodynamic interactions, watch for additive toxicity (see the earlier section "Additive effects" on page 26).
- When methadone or an interacting medication is taken intermittently, therapeutic levels will be difficult to maintain. Watch patients carefully for symptoms of opioid withdrawal or toxicity.
- Be aware that the use of illicit opioids or other drugs may influence patient symptoms. In the case of a relapse to drug use, take care not to misinterpret such symptoms as the results of other drug interactions.
- When starting methadone in a patient already being prescribed an interacting medication, simply titrate the methadone dose to the desired clinical effects.
- When starting, changing the dose of or discontinuing an interacting medication for a patient already in MMT, watch for increased or decreased methadone effects.
- If a patient's methadone dose had been adjusted because of an interaction, gradually resume the original dose after the interacting medication is stopped.

Note that the side-effects of other medications may mimic methadone withdrawal.

RESEARCH FINDINGS AND CLINICAL TIPS FOR SPECIFIC INTERACTIONS

The remainder of this chapter presents information about specific drug interactions with methadone.

Medications that can precipitate withdrawal

The following medications are contraindicated in MMT patients because they can precipitate withdrawal:

- opioid antagonists:
  - naltrexone (ReVia)
- partial agonist/mixed agonist-antagonists:
  - buprenorphine (Buprenex, Subutex, Suboxone)
  - butorphanol (Stadol NS)
  - nalbuphine (Nubain)
  - pentazocine (Talwin)

Medications that can change plasma levels of methadone

The two tables that follow on pages 28 to 36 summarize known information about drugs that interact with methadone by either *decreasing* its plasma levels (Table 4-1) or *increasing* these levels (Table 4-2).

Other interactions with methadone

A number of medications that have demonstrated, or been tested for, other interactions with methadone are listed in Table 4-3 on pages 36 to 38, together with the relevant findings and clinical tips.

Food interactions

The only significant known food interaction for methadone is with grapefruit juice. Its bioflavinoids have been reported to inhibit CYP3A4. Theoretically, there is a potential for elevated plasma levels of methadone. The clinical importance of this is unknown, however.

There is no evidence that orange juice causes the same effect.

Summary

Overall, methadone has more benefits than risks to both individuals and society. It must, however, be prescribed by those who appreciate the unique pharmacology of this very potent medication to prevent unintended adverse events (Peng et al., 2005).

TABLE 4-1

Medications that can decrease plasma levels of methadone

MEDICATION	FINDINGS	CLINICAL TIPS
Abacavir	In a study of 19 patients in MMT, there was a 34% decrease in peak concentration of abacavir and a 67% decrease in time to reach peak abacavir concentration, possibly because of the effect of methadone on gut motility. The clinical importance of this finding is unclear. One study showed that abacavir increased methadone clearance by 22%, which was not considered clinically relevant for most patients.	The combination of abacavir and methadone appears to be safe.
Amprenavir See also Amprenavir in Table 4-3.	Decreased methadone levels have been reported. No withdrawal symptoms have been reported.	Monitor MMT patients for possible withdrawal symptoms.
Barbiturates (phenobarbital, secobarbital, butalbital, etc.)	Enhanced methadone metabolism occurs via CYP3A4. May result in methadone withdrawal symptoms when a barbiturate is started in a patient stabilized on methadone, and may result in methadone intoxication when discontinued.	Monitor for withdrawal symptoms and adjust methadone dose accordingly when starting or stopping barbiturates. Where appropriate, consider alternatives to barbiturates.

Continued on next page

TABLE 4-1 MEDICATIONS THAT CAN DECREASE PLASMA LEVELS OF METHADONE (continued)

MEDICATION	FINDINGS	CLINICAL TIPS
Carbamazepine	Enhanced methadone metabolism occurs via CYP3A4. Enhanced hepatic metabolism of methadone may occur when starting carbamazepine in an MMT patient. This can result in withdrawal symptoms, necessitating an increase in methadone dose.	When discontinuing carbamazepine, decrease methadone dose accordingly. If appropriate, consider the use of valproic acid or gabapentin (neither of which affects CYP3A4 metabolism) as alternatives.
Efavirenz	Efavirenz induces CYPA3A4 metabolism. In a series of 11 patients started on efavirenz, nine described symptoms of withdrawal necessitating dose increases in the range of 15 to 30 mg. Symptoms of methadone withdrawal are reported to occur approximately eight days after starting efavirenz.	Be sure to distinguish the neurological side-effects of efavirenz, which occur during the first five days of treatment, from methadone withdrawal symptoms, which occur later. Monitor for withdrawal symptoms and adjust methadone dose when indicated.
Ethanol (chronic use)	Chronic use of alcohol can enhance hepatic metabolism of methadone through enzyme induction. Heavy users may experience opioid withdrawal symptoms after prolonged drinking. MMT patients should be warned about the effects of acute and chronic alcohol intake.	For information on acute use, see Ethanol in Table 4-2.
Lopinavir	The combination of ritonavir and lopinavir may decrease methadone levels.	Adjust methadone dose if necessary.
Nelfinavir	In vitro, nelfinavir appears to inhibit CYP3A4, but reports indicate decreased levels of methadone. In a study involving 14 patients being prescribed methadone, mean methadone peak concentration decreased by 43% and AUC decreased by 40%, yet none of the patients reported withdrawal symptoms or needed a dosage adjustment.	Monitor MMT patients for withdrawal symptoms and adjust methadone dose if necessary.

Continued on next page

TABLE 4-1 MEDICATIONS THAT CAN DECREASE PLASMA LEVELS OF METHADONE (continued)

MEDICATION	FINDINGS	CLINICAL TIPS
Nevirapine	Nevirapine induces CYP3A4 metabolism. Symptoms of methadone withdrawal have been reported to occur seven to 10 days after starting nevirapine.	Monitor MMT patients for withdrawal symptoms and adjust methadone dose as needed.
Phenytoin	Phenytoin enhances hepatic microsomal enzyme metabolism of methadone. When an MMT patient starts phenytoin, symptoms of methadone withdrawal may occur after a few days of treatment. Decreased plasma levels by 50% after three or four days of treatment have been reported.	Consider other treatment options if possible (valproic acid or gabapentin). If a patient must be maintained on both phenytoin and methadone, monitor and observe for symptoms. Adjust methadone dose if necessary when starting, increasing, decreasing or stopping phenytoin. Compliance with phenytoin treatment is important for maintaining therapeutic plasma levels of both phenytoin and methadone.
Primidone	Primidone is known to stimulate hepatic microsomal enzyme activity; this may result in decreased methadone levels.	Consider an alternative if possible.
Rifampin	Rifampin stimulates hepatic metabolism of methadone and induces some drug transporter proteins, such as P-glycoprotein. When rifampin is initiated in MMT patients, some may develop symptoms of opioid withdrawal within the first week of treatment and require an increase in methadone dose.	When rifampin is discontinued, monitor MMT patients for excessive methadone and decrease dose accordingly. Consider rifabutin (which does not stimulate microsomal enzymes) as an alternative.
Risperidone	Methadone withdrawal symptoms have been reported in one case.	

Continued on next page

TABLE 4-1 MEDICATIONS THAT CAN DECREASE PLASMA LEVELS OF METHADONE (continued)

MEDICATION	FINDINGS	CLINICAL TIPS
Ritonavir	Ritonavir appears to reduce methadone activity, possibly by induction of enzymes other than CYP3A4 or by affecting a P-glycoprotein system involved in access to the CNS, resulting in decreased methadone plasma levels. This interaction may be dependent on the dose of ritonavir. Previously it was predicted that ritonavir would increase methadone levels due to inhibition of CYP3A4. Case reports have shown the opposite. The combination of ritonavir and saquinavir is reported to induce methadone metabolism. One study showed a 37% decrease in AUC, but this was not associated with any evidence of opioid withdrawal symptoms. Further study suggests that the decrease in AUC may be the result of protein binding displacement. The combination of ritonavir and lopinavir may decrease methadone levels.	When combining ritonavir and saquinavir with methadone, monitor for symptoms of withdrawal. Methadone dose adjustment may or may not be needed. Consider indinavir, which does not interact with methadone, as an alternative option when appropriate. Observe patients taking a combination of ritonavir and lopinavir and adjust methadone dose as necessary.
Somatostatin	There has been one report of a patient treated with methadone for pain who, when started on somatostatin, experienced a diminished analgesic effect. The somatostatin analog octreotide may have a similar effect.	The clinical importance is unclear.
St. John's Wort	This herb is reported to induce CYP3A4 isoenzyme activity. In one report, of four patients taking St. John's Wort, two reported symptoms suggestive of withdrawal.	Monitor for symptoms of opioid withdrawal and increase methadone dose if needed, or consider a prescribed antidepressant.
Urinary acidifiers (ascorbic acid [vitamin C], ammonium chloride, potassium phosphate, sodium phosphate)	Urinary acidifiers may increase methadone elimination, resulting in reduced plasma methadone concentrations and possible opioid withdrawal symptoms.	The clinical importance is unclear.

TABLE 4-2

Medications that can increase plasma levels of methadone

MEDICATION	FINDINGS	CLINICAL TIPS
Amitriptyline	There are reports of MMT patients using amitriptyline to enhance the psychoactive effects of methadone.	
Benzodiazepines See also Diazepam.	All benzodiazepines can be problematic for MMT patients due to dependence liability and the risk of overdose related to additive toxicity. Benzodiazepines may contribute to deaths from methadone toxicity by increasing obstruction of the upper respiratory system. Benzodiazepine dependence is related to poor outcomes in MMT.	Exercise extreme caution when combining opioids and benzodiazepines.
Cimetidine	Cimetidine is an inhibitor of CYP3A4 and increases methadone levels. The clinical importance is unclear.	Consider ranitidine as an alternative.
Ciprofloxacin	Ciprofloxacin is an inhibitor of CYP3A4 metabolism. Profound sedation, confusion and respiratory distress (reversed by naloxone treatment) have been reported.	Monitor MMT patients carefully for symptoms of methadone overdose. Consider decreasing methadone dose while a patient is on ciprofloxacin (and increasing it correspondingly when ciprofloxacin is discontinued). Alternatively, consider using another antibiotic instead.
Clarithromycin	Clarithromycin inhibits CYP3A4. Theoretically, clarithromycin may increase methadone levels. The clinical importance is unclear.	Monitor for sedation and other symptoms of opioid toxicity.
Delavirdine	Delavirdine inhibits CYP3A4. Although there are no studies to confirm this, methadone levels may be increased.	Monitor for methadone toxicity.

Continued on next page

TABLE 4-2: MEDICATIONS THAT CAN INCREASE PLASMA LEVELS OF METHADONE (continued)

MEDICATION	FINDINGS	CLINICAL TIPS
Diazepam	Diazepam is metabolized by CYP3A4. Enhanced psychoactive effects, similar to those produced by short-acting opioids when taken shortly before or after methadone, have been reported. All benzodiazepines can be problematic for MMT patients due to dependence liability and the risk of overdose related to additive toxicity. Benzodiazepines may contribute to deaths from methadone toxicity by increasing obstruction of the upper respiratory system. Benzodiazepine dependence is related to poor outcomes in MMT.	Exercise extreme caution when combining opioids and benzodiazepines.
Disulfiram	Disulfiram may decrease methadone metabolism. This is not clinically significant.	
Erythromycins (including clarithromycin)	Erythromycins inhibit CYP3A4. Theoretically, this may increase methadone levels. The clinical importance is unclear.	Monitor for sedation and other symptoms of opioid toxicity. Although no data are currently available, azithromycin (which does not affect CYP3A4) may be considered as an alternative.
Ethanol (acute use)	Acute high blood alcohol concentrations reduce methadone metabolism by competing for metabolic enzyme activity.	Observe patient for opioid toxicity and overdose. For effects of chronic alcohol intake, see Ethanol in Table 4-1.

Continued on next page

TABLE 4-2: MEDICATIONS THAT CAN INCREASE PLASMA LEVELS OF METHADONE (continued)

MEDICATION	FINDINGS	CLINICAL TIPS
Fluconazole	Fluconazole inhibits CYP3A4. Respiratory depression has been reported in one patient after two days of fluconazole administration. In a series of 35 patients started on fluconazole, increased methadone levels (35% increase in AUC) were observed after 14 days of treatment. Patients reported no symptoms and there were no methadone dose adjustments. Itraconazole may affect methadone levels in a similar manner.	Observe MMT patients for opioid toxicity and reduce methadone dose as required. If appropriate, consider terbinafine (which does not inhibit CYP3A4) as an alternative antifungal agent.
Fluoxetine	Fluoxetine is a weak inhibitor of CYP3A4. No adverse consequences were reported in a study of 44 MMT patients initiated on fluoxetine. Another study of nine MMT patients showed a minimal increase in methadone levels.	Although the clinical importance is unclear, monitor for increased methadone effects and reduce methadone dose if needed.
Fluvoxamine	Fluvoxamine is a potent inhibitor of CYP3A4; it can also inhibit CYP1A2 and CYP2C19. This drug can increase methadone levels (varying from 20% to 100%). In one case report, an MMT patient on a stable dose of methadone (70 mg) was started on fluvoxamine (100 mg per day) and then was admitted to hospital after three weeks with respiratory depression.	If fluvoxamine is started for patients in MMT, monitor carefully for opioid toxicity (e.g., sedation, respiratory depression) and decrease methadone dose as needed. Although there are no studies comparing them, if appropriate, consider citalopram or venlafaxine as alternatives because they have little or no effect on CYP3A4.
Indinavir	No interaction with methadone has been reported. In a series of 12 MMT patients initiated on indinavir, there were no reported effects on methadone levels.	

Continued on next page

TABLE 4-2: MEDICATIONS THAT CAN INCREASE PLASMA LEVELS OF METHADONE (continued)

MEDICATION	FINDINGS	CLINICAL TIPS
Itraconazole	Itraconazole may affect methadone levels in a manner similar to fluconazole. In a series of 35 patients started on fluconazole, increased methadone levels (35% increase in AUC) were observed after 14 days of treatment. Patients reported no symptoms and there were no methadone dose adjustments.	
Ketoconazole	Ketoconazole inhibits CYP3A4. It may decrease methadone metabolism, resulting in increased methadone effects.	Monitor MMT patients for opioid intoxication (e.g., sedation or respiratory depression) and decrease methadone dose as necessary. If appropriate, consider the use of terbinafine (which does not inhibit CYP3A4) as an alternative treatment option.
Nefazodone	Nefazodone is a potent CYP3A4 inhibitor. It may increase plasma levels of methadone.	Monitor MMT patients for symptoms of opioid intoxication and decrease methadone dose if needed.
Paroxetine	Paroxetine is a potent CYP2D6 inhibitor and a mild inhibitor of CYP3A4, CYP2C9 and CYP2C19. In a series of 10 MMT patients, paroxetine (20 mg per day) significantly increased methadone plasma levels (from 32% to 83%). Patients reported no symptoms. The wide variation may be the result of differences in genetic predisposition (i.e., extensive versus poor metabolizers of CYP2D6).	Monitor MMT patients for symptoms of opioid intoxication and adjust methadone dose as needed.

Continued on next page

TABLE 4-2: MEDICATIONS THAT CAN INCREASE PLASMA LEVELS OF METHADONE (continued)

MEDICATION	FINDINGS	CLINICAL TIPS
Saquinavir	No interaction has been reported to date. The combination of ritonavir and saquinavir is reported to induce methadone metabolism. One study showed a 37% decrease in AUC, but this was not associated with any evidence of opioid withdrawal symptoms. Further study suggests that the decrease in AUC may be the result of protein binding displacement.	When combining ritonavir and saquinavir with methadone, monitor patient for symptoms of withdrawal. Methadone dose adjustment may not be needed.
Sertraline	A study involving 31 depressed MMT patients suggests that sertraline may produce a modest increase in methadone levels over the first six weeks of treatment, with return to baseline after six weeks.	Watch for increased methadone effects during the first six weeks after starting sertraline. Decrease methadone dose if needed.
Urinary alkalizers	Theoretically, urinary alkalizers may increase renal reabsorption of methadone.	

TABLE 4-3

Effects of methadone on pharmacokinetics of other medications

MEDICATION	FINDINGS	CLINICAL TIPS
Abacavir	In a study of 19 patients in MMT, there was a 34% decrease in peak concentration of abacavir and a 67% decrease in time to reach peak abacavir concentration, possibly because of the effect of methadone on gut motility. The clinical importance is unclear. One study showed that abacavir increased methadone clearance by 22%, which was not considered clinically relevant for most patients.	The combination of abacavir and methadone appears to be safe.

Continued on next page

TABLE 4-3: EFFECTS OF METHADONE ON PHARMACOKINETICS OF OTHER MEDICATIONS (continued)

MEDICATION	FINDINGS	CLINICAL TIPS
Amprenavir	Amprenavir may be less effective in MMT patients because of decreased plasma concentrations. Co-administration of methadone and amprenavir resulted in a 30%, 27% and 25% decrease in serum aprenavir AUC, C_{max} and C_{min}, respectively.	Alternative anti-retroviral therapy may be considered.
Desipramine	It has been shown that plasma concentration of desipramine increases in patients taking methadone. The possible mechanism for this is reduced hydroxylation of desipramine.	Monitor plasma levels of desipramine and observe for desipramine toxicity. It may be necessary to adjust the desipramine dose.
Didanosine	Methadone decreased AUC for didanosine by 60% and C_{max} by 64%. The possible mechanism is a delay in gastric motility caused by methadone. An enteric-coated didanosine formulation did not appear to be affected by methadone and may not require a dose change.	An increase in didanosine dose may be indicated, or another formulation should be considered.
Monoamine oxidase inhibitors (MAOIs, including moclobemide, phenelzine and tranylcypromine)	There are no reports of interactions with methadone. Non-selective MAOIs with concurrent use of meperidine resulted in death. Morphine–MAOI interactions have been less severe than meperidine–MAOI interactions.	Use extreme caution, or avoid combining MAOIs and opioids.
Nifedipine	Methadone can inhibit oxidation of nifedipine in vitro, which may result in greater-than-expected nifedipine effects or nifedipine toxicity. The clinical significance is unclear.	

Continued on next page

TABLE 4-3: EFFECTS OF METHADONE ON PHARMACOKINETICS OF OTHER MEDICATIONS (continued)

MEDICATION	FINDINGS	CLINICAL TIPS
Stavudine	Decreased stavudine AUC of 18% and C_{max} of 39% have been reported. The clinical importance is unclear.	
Zidovudine (AZT)	In a series of eight patients in MMT, oral zidovudine levels increased by 29% and intravenous zidovudine levels increased by 41%. This interaction does not seem to occur with buprenorphine. Methadone inhibits zidovudine glucuronidation and may increase the formation of zidovudine's metabolite, which is thought to produce anemia.	MMT patients may be at increased risk for zidovudine side-effects and toxicity, including headache, nausea and vomiting. It is important not to confuse these side-effects with methadone withdrawal. Monitor MMT patients for increased zidovudine toxicity. Reduce zidovudine dose as necessary.

References

Al-Adwani A. & Basu N. (2004). Methadone and excessive sweating. *Addiction, 99*, 259.

Antoniou, T. & Tseng, A.L. (2002). Interactions between recreational drugs and antiretroviral agents. *Annals of Pharmacotherapy, 36*, 1598–1613.

Atkinson, R.L. (1987). Opioid regulation of food intake and body weight in humans. *Federation Proceedings, 46*, 178–182.

Baselt, R.C. (2000). *Disposition of Toxic Drugs and Chemicals in Man* (5th ed.). Foster City, CA: Chemical Toxicity Institute.

Begré, S., von Bardeleben, U., Ladewig, D., Jaquet-Rochat, S., Cosendai-Savary, L. & Golay, K.P. (2002). Paroxetine increases steady-state concentrations of (R)-methadone in CYP2D6 extensive but not poor metabolizers. *Journal of Clinical Psychopharmacology, 22* (2), 211–215.

Bertz, R.J. & Granneman, G.R. (1997). Use of in vitro and in vivo data to estimate the likelihood of metabolic pharmacokinetic interactions. *Clinical Pharmacokinetics, 32* (3), 210–256.

Bogucka-Bonikowska, A., Baran-Furga, H., Chmielewska, K, Habrat, B., Scinska, A., Kukwa, A. et al. (2002). Taste function in methadone-maintained opioid-dependent men. *Drug and Alcohol Dependence, 68* (1), 113–117.

Brown, R., Balousek, S., Mundt, M. & Fleming, M. (2005). Methadone maintenance and male sexual dysfunction. *Journal of Addictive Diseases, 24*, 91–106.

Caflisch, C., Figner, B. & Eich, D. (2003). Biperiden for excessive sweating from methadone. *American Journal of Psychiatry, 160*, 386–387.

Crowley, T.J. & Simpson, R. (1978). Methadone dose and human sexual behaviour. *International Journal of the Addictions, 13*, 285–295.

Dalton, M.S. & Duncan, D.W. (1979). Fifty opiate addicts treated with methadone blockade—eight year follow-up. *Medical Journal of Australia, 1*, 153–154.

Daniell, H.W. (2002). Hypogonadism in men consuming sustained-action oral opioids. *Journal of Pain, 3*, 377–384.

Darke, S., Sims, J., McDonald, S. & Wickes, W. (2000). Cognitive impairment among methadone maintenance patients. *Addiction, 95* (5), 687–695.

Davis, M.P. & Walsh, D. (2001). Methadone for relief of cancer pain: A review of pharmacokinetics, pharmacodynamics, drug interactions and protocols of administration. *Supportive Care in Cancer, 9* (2), 73–83.

Dole, V.P., Foldes, F.F., Trigg, H., Robinson, J.W. & Blatman, S. (1973). Methadone poisoning: Diagnosis and treatment. In C.D. Chambers (Ed.), *Methadone: Experiences and Issues* (pp. 177–182). New York: Brill Leon Behavioural Publications.

Doverty, M., Somogyi, A.A., White, J.M., Bochner, F., Beare, C.H. & Menelaou, A. (2001). Methadone maintenance patients are cross-tolerant to the antinociceptive effects of morphine. *Pain, 93,* 155–163.

Doverty, M., White, J.M., Somogyi, A.A., Bochner, F., Ali, R. & Ling, W. (2001). Hyperalgesic responses in methadone maintenance patients. *Pain, 90,* 91–96.

Evans, L.E., Swainson, C.P., Roscoe, P. & Prescott, L.F. (1973). Treatment of drug overdosage with naloxone, a specific narcotic antagonist. *The Lancet, 1,* 452–455.

Fainsinger, R., Schoeller, T. & Bruera, E. (1993). Methadone in the management of cancer pain: A review. *Pain, 52,* 137–147.

Foster, D.J., Somogyi, A.A., Dyer, K.R., White, J.M. & Bochner, F. (2000). Steady-state pharmacokinetics of (R)- and (S)-methadone in methadone maintenance patients. *British Journal of Clinical Pharmacology, 50* (5), 427–440.

Fuller, M.A. & Sajatovic, M. (2001). *Drug Information for Mental Health.* Hudson, OH: Lexi-Comp.

Garriott, J.C., Sturner, W.Q. & Mason, M.F. (1973). Toxicological findings in six fatalities involving methadone. *Clinical Toxicology, 6,* 163–173.

Hallinan, R., Byrne, A., Agho, K., McMahon, C.G., Tynan, P. & Attia, J. (2007). Hypogonadism in men receiving methadone and buprenorphine maintenance treatment. *International Journal of Andrology* [OnlineEarly article], doi:10.1111/j.1365-2605.2007.00824.x.

Harding-Pink, D. (1993). Methadone: One person's maintenance dose is another's poison. *The Lancet, 341* (8846), 665–666.

Kolarzyk, E., Chrostek Maj, J., Pach, D., Janik, A., Kwiatkowski, J. & Szurkowska, M. (2005). Assessment of daily nutrition ratios of opiate-dependent persons before and after 4 years of methadone maintenance treatment. *Przeglad Lekarski, 62* (6), 368–372.

Kolarzyk, E., Jenner, B., Szpanowska-Wohn, A., Pach, D. & Szurkowska, M. (2005). The changes in taste preferences during 4-year period of methadone maintenance treatment. *Przeglad Lekarski, 62* (6), 378–381.

Kolarzyk, E., Pach, D., Wojtowicz, B., Szpanowska-Wohn, A. & Szurkowska, M. (2005). Nutritional status of the opiate dependent persons after 4 years of methadone maintenance treatment. *Przeglad Lekarski, 62* (6), 373-387.

Krantz, M.J., Lewkowiez, L., Hays, H., Woodroffe, M.A., Robertson, A.D. & Mehler, P.S. (2002). Torsade de pointes associated with very-high-dose methadone. *Annals of Internal Medicine, 137* (6), 501–504.

Krantz, M.J., Lowery, C.M., Martell, B.A., Gourevitch, M.N. & Arnsten J.H. (2005). Effects of methadone on QT-interval dispersion. *Pharmacotherapy, 25* (11), 1523-1529.

Krantz, M.J. & Mehler, P.S. (2003). Synthetic opioids and QT prolongation. *Archives of Internal Medicine, 163,* 1615.

Langman M.J. (2001). Ulcer complications associated with anti-inflammatory drug use. What is the extent of the disease burden? *Pharmacoepidemiology and Drug Safety, 10* (1), 13-19.

Lawlor, P.G. (2002). The panorama of opioid-related cognitive dysfunction in patients with cancer: A critical literature appraisal. *Cancer, 94* (6), 1836–1853.

Lugo, R.A., Satterfield, K.L. & Kern, S.E. (2005). Pharmacokinetics of methadone. *Journal of Pain and Palliative Care Pharmacotherapy, 19,* 13–24.

Lyvers, M. & Yakimoff, M. (2003). Neuropsychological correlates of opioid dependence and withdrawal. *Addictive Behaviors, 28* (3), 605–611.

Martell, B.A., Arnsten, J.H., Ray, B. & Gourevitch, M.N. (2003). The impact of methadone induction on cardiac conduction in opiate users. *Annals of Internal Medicine, 139,* 154–155.

McLellan, A.T. (1983). Patient characteristics associated with outcome. In J.R. Cooper, F. Altman, B.S. Brown & D. Czechowicz (Eds.), *Research on the Treatment of Narcotic Addiction: State of the Art* (pp. 500–529). NIDA Monograph Series. Rockville, MD: National Institute of Drug Abuse Treatment.

Mintzer, M.Z. & Stitzer, M.L. (2002). Cognitive impairment in methadone maintenance patients. *Drug and Alcohol Dependence, 67* (1), 41–51.

Moolchan, E.T., Umbricht, A. & Epstein, D. (2001). Therapeutic drug monitoring in methadone maintenance: Choosing a matrix. *Journal of Addictive Diseases, 20* (2), 55–73.

Nolan, L.J. & Scagnelli, L.M. (2007). Preference for sweet foods and higher body mass index in patients being treated in long-term methadone maintenance. *Substance Use and Misuse, 42* (10), 1555-1566.

O'Neill, W.M., Hanks, G.W., Simpson, P., Fallon, M.T., Jenkins, E. & Wesnes, K. (2000). The cognitive and psychomotor effects of morphine in healthy subjects: A randomized controlled trial of repeated (four) oral doses of dextropropoxyphene, morphine, lorazepam and placebo. *Pain, 85* (1–2), 209–215.

Peng, P.W., Tumber, P.S. & Gourlay, D. (2005). Review article: Perioperative pain management of patients on methadone therapy. *Canadian Journal of Anaesthesia, 52*, 513–523.

Pud, D., Cohen, D., Lawental, E. & Eisenberg, E. (2006). Opioids and abnormal pain perception: New evidence from a study of chronic opioid addicts and healthy subjects. *Drug and Alcohol Dependence, 82* (3), 218–223.

Quigley C. (2004). Opioid switching to improve pain relief and drug tolerability. Cochrane Database of Systematic Reviews, 3:CD004847.

Schindler, S., Ortner, R., Peternell, A., Eder, H., Opgenoorth, E. & Fischer, G. (2004). Maintenance therapy with synthetic opioids and driving aptitude. *European Addiction Research, 10* (2), 80–87.

Scholz, M. (2000). Managing constipation that's opioid-induced. *RN, 63*, 103.

Shir, Y., Rosen, G., Zeldin, A. & Davidson, E.M. (2001). Methadone is safe for treating hospitalized patients with severe pain. *Canadian Journal of Anaesthesia, 48*, 1109–1113.

Srivastava, A. & Kahan, M. (2006). Methadone induction doses: Are our current practices safe? *Journal of Addictive Diseases, 25* (3), 5–13.

Stimmel, B. (2003). Methadone and affairs of the heart and of the brain. *Journal of Addictive Diseases, 22* (3), 1–5.

Sullivan, H.R., Due, S.L. & McMahon R.E. (1972). The identification of three new metabolites of methadone in man and in the rat. *Journal of the American Chemical Society, 94* (11), 4050–4051.

Wang, J.S. & DeVane, C.L. (2003). Involvement of CYP3A4, CYP2C8, and CYP2D6 in the metabolism of (R)- and (S)-methadone in vitro. *Drug Metabolism and Disposition, 31* (6), 742–747.

World Health Organization (WHO), United Nations Office on Drugs and Crime (UNODC) & Joint United Nations Programme on HIV/AIDS (UNAIDS). (2004). *Substitution Maintenance Therapy in the Management of Opioid Dependence and HIV/AIDS Prevention*. [Position paper]. New York: Author.

Yuan, C.S., Foss, J.F., O'Connor, M., Moss, J. & Roizen, M.F. (1998). Gut motility and transit changes in patients receiving long-term methadone maintenance. *Journal of Clinical Pharmacology, 38*, 931–935.

SECTION II

Framework for methadone maintenance treatment

CHAPTER 5

Clinical diagnosis for MMT

This chapter discusses the indications for opioid dependence and provides guidelines for assessing the methadone patient prior to treatment.

Indications for methadone treatment

Clinicians must have a full understanding of the signs and symptoms of opioid withdrawal to successfully detect and diagnose opioid dependence.

Careful planning is extremely important when treating opioid dependence. Methadone should be reserved for those who meet the criteria for opioid dependence and have not responded to intensive treatment programs or are not suitable candidates for such treatment. Patients who meet the criteria for abuse but who are under 18 years of age, have been using for a short period of time, are using low- to medium-potency combination opioids (such as codeine or oxycodone) and/or are treatment-naive should not immediately be offered MMT. These individuals could benefit from withdrawal management and intensive outpatient or inpatient substance abuse treatment, treatment of any co-occurring mental health disorder such as depression, and/or involvement in mutual aid programs (such as Narcotics Anonymous or Cocaine nonymous), as well as from immunization and health education.

The management of opioid withdrawal is often the first step in deciding which treatment option is best for the patient.

Although MMT is considerably more effective than abstinence-based treatment, it is in most cases a long-term treatment that requires considerable effort and commitment on the patient's part. For this reason, methadone treatment is most clearly indicated for patients who have a long history of established opioid dependence and have been unsuccessful or are likely to be unsuccessful with abstinence-based treatments.

In cases where abstinence-based treatment is advised rather than methadone, patients should be warned that they run the risk of overdose due to loss of tolerance if they relapse. Follow-up should be arranged after completion of the treatment program so the patients can be offered methadone treatment should they relapse (Morrison, 2003).

The major factors to consider in determining the appropriateness of methadone treatment are summarized in Table 5-1 on page 44.

Assessing the MMT patient

Before starting a patient on MMT, a comprehensive medical assessment is essential, to formulate a treatment plan and identify potentially treatable medical, psychiatric and social problems.

SUBSTANCE USE

Physicians should document the amount, pattern and duration of the patient's opioid use, the route of administration and the time of last use.

Polysubstance abuse is common among opioid users; for example, benzodiazepines are commonly used to relieve opioid withdrawal symptoms, and many patients don't realize that the combination may pose significant risks during methadone titration. Therefore, it is necessary to also take a complete substance use history at baseline, including careful inquiry about alcohol, cocaine, sedatives, tobacco, methamphetamine and cannabis use.

Patients should also be asked if they have experienced any symptoms of opioid withdrawal, such as insomnia and myalgias.

TABLE 5-1

Factors affecting the decision to offer MMT

FACTOR	COMMENTS
Outcome of previous abstinence-based treatments	Patients who have repeatedly relapsed immediately after discharge from abstinence-based treatment programs should be considered for methadone treatment. However, if they had prolonged periods of abstinence following such programs, they might consider trying again.
Patient preference	Many patients are convinced that methadone is the best option for them. Others prefer to try abstinence first.
Amount of opioids used	Patients with chronic pain who are also dependent on moderate doses of weak opioids such as codeine might attempt "structured opioid therapy" first. In this therapy, sustained-release opioids are dispensed daily or several times per week by the pharmacy, and the patient provides regular urine drug screens. Structured opioid therapy is best for patients who acquire opioids only from one physician, do not crush, bite or inject their tablets, are not currently dependent on other drugs and have a genuine source of organic pain. Opioid-dependent patients who do not meet these criteria should be referred for abstinence-based or methadone treatment.
Age and duration of use	Adolescents who have been abusing opioids for only a few weeks or months might prefer abstinence-based treatment. If methadone treatment is initiated, tapering might be considered once the patient is stable and has re-engaged in school and family life.

PREVIOUS TREATMENT

The history of any previous treatment is also useful in planning the best approach for a patient. For example, repeated relapses following abstinence-based treatment programs confirm the need for methadone treatment. If a patient has received MMT in the past, the physician should obtain as much information as possible from the previous providers to determine how well the patient responded and what the reasons were for dropping out or discharge.

SOCIAL FACTORS

Social factors such as living arrangements, substance use among family members, parenting arrangements and the safety of children at home can affect treatment plans and outcomes. Substance use among family members especially may have a major impact on the patient's treatment and prognosis. Partners of substance users should be asked about physical abuse.

PSYCHIATRIC HISTORY

People who use opioids are at extremely high risk for suicide. Even those who do not have a pre-existing psychiatric disorder may experience thoughts of suicide because of the dysphoria associated with withdrawal and the serious personal difficulties that often accompany substance abuse. Usually the suicidal thoughts respond to supportive counselling or brief hospitalization for withdrawal management. Patients should also be assessed for concurrent mood, anxiety and psychotic disorders.

(For more on MMT and concurrent psychiatric illnesses, see Chapter 13, "MMT and concurrent psychiatric illness.")

HIGH-RISK BEHAVIOUR

High-risk behaviours are common, including unsafe sex, lack of contraception and needle sharing. Women should be asked about use of birth control and the possibility of pregnancy. Also note that in Ontario, physicians are required by law to report alcohol or other drug use and driving to the provincial Ministry of Transportation. (For more on MMT and driving, see Chapter 17, "Methadone and driving.")

PHYSICAL EXAM

Special attention should be given to signs of opioid withdrawal, malnutrition, jaundice, epatosplenomegaly, cardiovascular and respiratory status, pupil size, needle tracks and abscesses. The general demeanour of the patient should be assessed: an individual who is in withdrawal will appear uncomfortable and restless. The patient should be examined for signs of autonomic hyperactivity, including dilated pupils, tachycardia, hypertension, goosebumps, tremor, sweating, yawning, lacrimation and active bowel sounds. (For details on assessing physical withdrawal, see Table 10-1, "Short Opiate Withdrawal Scale" (SOWS), in Chapter 10.)

LABORATORY TESTS

Baseline laboratory tests include CBC, MCV and GGT (to detect heavy alcohol consumption), AST, ALT (viral or alcoholic hepatitis), serology for hepatitis B and C and for HIV, and B-HCG for women in the reproductive age group. At least one urine drug screen (see Chapter 8) must be completed during the assessment phase, and the results must be interpreted before the patient begins MMT.

Assessment summary

A checklist summarizing the items to be covered in assessing a patient at the start of MMT is presented in Table 5-2.

TABLE 5-2

Methadone patient assessment checklist

HISTORY

- amount, pattern and route of opioid use
- withdrawal symptoms
- other drug use (alcohol, cocaine, tobacco, methamphetamine, benzodiazepines, cannabis)
- consequences of use (physical, social, occupational, legal, financial)
- social situation, including safety of children living at home
- depression, anxiety, psychosis, suicidal ideation
- spouse or child abuse
- previous treatment attempts
- in the case of injection drug use: sharing of injection equipment; history of hepatitis B or C and/or HIV
- high-risk sexual activity (involvement in the sex trade or engaging in sexual activity while impaired)
- possibility of pregnancy

PHYSICAL

- track marks
- liver, spleen, cardiovascular
- respiratory

LABORATORY

- CBC, MCV, CGT
- AST, ALT
- β-HCG
- hepatitis B and C, HIV
- urine drug screen

Reference

Morrison, C.L. (2003). Loss of tolerance and overdose mortality with detoxification: Deaths have been associated with interventions. *British Medical Journal, 327* (7411), 393.

CHAPTER 6

Abstinence-based interventions for opioid withdrawal

If abstinence-based treatment is chosen (because MMT is deemed not appropriate, or is not desired or not available), treatment of opioid withdrawal is a necessary first step. This chapter explains various interventions for managing such withdrawal, including tapering with methadone, tapering with prescription opioids and using clonidine.

Management of opioid withdrawal

GENERAL PRINCIPLES

Management of withdrawal should always be combined with enrolment in a drug rehabilitation program. Regardless of the treatment protocol, managed withdrawal alone usually does not result in long-term abstinence (Amato et al., 2004). Furthermore, paradoxically, managed withdrawal carries a significant risk of overdose on relapse. This is because patients who have been abstinent for a week or longer have lost much of their tolerance to opioids, and they may overdose if they relapse to their usual opioid dose. Psychosocial support from friends and families is extremely important.

Inpatient admission should be considered for opioid-dependent patients who are medically ill, have been unsuccessful with outpatient withdrawal management or are about to be admitted to a rehabilitation program that does not accept patients on methadone. There may also be psychiatric or psychosocial reasons for considering inpatient admission.

OVERVIEW OF INTERVENTIONS

Physicians have several intervention options for helping their patients cope with opioid withdrawal. The following therapies are commonly used for opioid withdrawal in Canada:

- tapering doses of methadone
- tapering doses of prescription opioids
- clonidine.

In all cases it is advisable to provide the following types of symptomatic pharmacological treatments:

- an antiemetic (e.g., dimenhydrinate [50 mg po q6h prn]) for nausea and vomiting)
- an NSAID (e.g., ibuprofen [200–400 mg po qid prn]) for muscle, joint or back pain
- an antidiarrheal agent (e.g., loperamide [2 mg po after each loose stool to a maximum 8 mg per 24 hours]).

Physicians may choose to prescribe a short course of benzodiazepines to relieve insomnia in patients undergoing opioid withdrawal. This approach should be undertaken with caution, however, because sedative abuse and dependence are common among people who are opioid dependent. Trazodone is a safe alternative to benzodiazepines.

Patients in managed withdrawal need a supportive environment that includes adequate oral hydration, warm clothing and blankets for chills, hot baths, supportive and encouraging caregivers and, most importantly, the absence of any cues for drug use.

MANAGING OPIOID WITHDRAWAL USING CLONIDINE

Clonidine has been shown to be more effective than placebo in suppressing symptoms of withdrawal from opioids (Jasinski et al., 1985); however, controlled trials suggest that it is probably less effective than methadone (San et al., 1990).

Suggested protocol for using clonidine in managing opioid withdrawal

Clonidine is thought to act by central inhibition of the hypernoradrenergic state that occurs in opioid withdrawal. For outpatients, a test dose of clonidine 0.1 mg should be given. If the patient's blood pressure remains above 90/60 mm Hg after one hour, an initial dose of 0.1 mg tid–qid may be prescribed. If necessary, this may be increased to 0.2 mg tid–qid prn the following day, although the risk of symptomatic hypotension increases with this dose. After the first five or six days, clonidine may be used on an as-needed basis.

If clonidine has been used daily for two weeks or more, it should be tapered rather than simply stopped; abrupt discontinuation can cause rebound hypertension.

Side-effects

The side-effects of clonidine include postural hypotension, sedation and dry mouth. Patients should be advised to avoid prolonged hot baths, as they can lead to venous pooling and hypotension. Patients should also be advised not to drive motor vehicles if they find that clonidine induces drowsiness.

Patients taking moderate or high doses of clonidine should be clearly warned that they risk life-threatening hypotension should they inject opioids.

Clondine should be used with caution in patients who have underlying heart disease or who are on anti-hypertensive medications.

Inpatient treatment for larger doses

For inpatients, whose blood pressure and sedation can be monitored more closely, clonidine doses of 0.2 to 0.3 mg orally every four hours can be administered up to a daily maximum of 2.0 mg. The dose should be withheld if the patient is symptom-free or if his or her blood pressure is less than 90/60 mm Hg.

MANAGING INPATIENT WITHDRAWAL USING METHADONE

The in-hospital provision of methadone can help convince an opioid-dependent patient to stay in hospital and complete treatment; however, methadone should only be titrated by an experienced methadone prescriber. Methadone can be dangerous when given to acutely ill patients, particularly if they have respiratory compromise or decreased level of consciousness, or they are on multiple medications. Benzodiazepines should not be used during titration.

On the first full day of admission, methadone is given as a morning dose of 10 to 20 mg, followed by no more than two prn doses of 5 mg q6h. Nurses should be educated about opioid withdrawal symptoms and advised to hold the methadone and contact the physician if the patient appears drowsy. On the second day of admission, the total dose for the first 24-hour period is dispensed as a single dose, with one or two 5-mg prn doses added. In this manner the dose is increased daily by 5 to 10 mg until a dose of 40 to 80 mg is reached.

If the patient is not going on to receive maintenance treatment, the dose is then tapered by 5 to 10 mg per day.

(See Chapter 7 for a more complete description of dosing guidelines and the risks associated with the first two weeks of methadone treatment.)

Temporary licence to supervise inpatient opioid withdrawal

In Canada, physicians may obtain a temporary licence to prescribe methadone in a hospital setting from the Office of Controlled Substances (613 946-5139).

MANAGING OUTPATIENT WITHDRAWAL USING METHADONE

The general principles of methadone dosing, as outlined in Chapter 7, apply to outpatient withdrawal management as well as to MMT:

- begin with a safe initial dose of 15 to 30 mg for the first three days
- titrate upward by 10 to 15 mg every three to five days.

Once the optimal dose is reached, it should be tapered by no more than 2 to 5 mg at a time. The rate of the taper should be determined by the completion date agreed to by physician and patient, as well as the patient's symptoms and drug use. The taper might need to be slowed when the dose reaches 20 mg. In general, reductions of 10 per cent per day of the daily dose are not perceived by the patient.

Outpatient tapering often takes six months or more; slow tapers work better than rapid tapers. A patient who originally chose to undergo managed withdrawal rather than enter MMT should have the option of choosing to enter maintenance treatment at any time during the taper. Counselling and urine drug screening should continue throughout the taper.

TAPERING OUTPATIENTS USING OPIOIDS OTHER THAN METHADONE

Buprenorphine, which is now available in Canada in combination with naloxone under the brand name Suboxone, may turn out to be an ideal agent for outpatient tapers. It has several advantages:

- the optimal dose can be reached within days
- its withdrawal syndrome is milder than that of methadone
- it has a very low risk of overdose.

Other than buprenorphine, opioid tapering may be useful for patients dependent on milder opioid analgesics such as codeine. For example, a patient taking 20 tablets of Tylenol 1 daily could safely and conveniently begin a taper with 50 to 100 mg bid of Codeine Contin or four tablets a day of Tylenol 3.

Outpatient tapering with opioids other than methadone or buprenorphine should not be attempted unless all three of the following criteria are present:

- there is a possibility that the patient might have an organic source of pain requiring opioid therapy
- the physician has a long-standing relationship with the patient and is confident that the risk of diversion or acquiring opioids from other sources is minimal
- the patient gives consent to contact other physicians and pharmacists who have been involved in the patient's care.

Physicians should avoid tapering with the opioid on which the patient has become dependent. If possible they should also avoid oxycodone and hydromorphone, because they have high abuse liabilities.

Daily, twice-weekly or weekly dispensing of the medication is recommended. Urine drug screening is advised, although it will only detect double-doctoring if the patient uses a different opioid from the one prescribed for the managed withdrawal.

The physician should set a target date of two to six months for completion of the taper. Patients should be referred to a drug rehabilitation program and possibly an addiction specialist and pain specialist.

"RAPID OPIOID DETOXIFICATION"

Benefits and risks

In combination with general anesthesia, the "rapid opioid detoxification"[1] protocol aims to allow people dependent on opioids to undergo managed withdrawal over a 24-hour period without experiencing the adverse symptoms of withdrawal. One case series found that 50 per cent of patients undergoing "rapid opioid detoxification" were abstinent at six months (Albanese et al., 2000); however, there is little evidence that the treatment is superior to other forms of medically managed withdrawal. Deaths have been reported due to the procedure itself, and to overdose following relapse to opioid use (Hamilton et al., 2002; San et al., 1995).

In a more recent well-designed study in the United States, there was little evidence of benefit from "rapid opioid detoxification" (Collins et al., 2005). This study was done on 106 treatment-seeking, heroin-dependent patients between the ages of 21 and 50. Each was randomly assigned to one of three groups for the first 72 hours:

- anesthesia-assisted "rapid opioid detoxification" with naltrexone induction
- buprenorphine-assisted "rapid opioid detoxification" with naltrexone induction, or
- clonidine-assisted "rapid opioid detoxification" with delayed naltrexone induction.

All groups subsequently received 12 weeks of outpatient naltrexone maintenance with relapse prevention psychotherapy. Patients were healthy, without comorbid psychiatric or substance use disorders. Induction onto

1 "Rapid opioid detoxification" should not be confused with withdrawal management. In this context the term "detoxification" is used, consistent with research literature, only when referring to "rapid opioid detoxification."

naltrexone occurred in only 21 per cent of those undergoing clonidine-assisted detoxification, whereas 94 per cent of the anesthesia-assisted group and 97 per cent of the buprenorphine-assisted group were inducted onto naltrexone; however, there were no differences in the rates of completion of inpatient detoxification. Treatment retention over 12 weeks was not significantly different among the groups, although the clonidine group fared the worst. The anesthesia procedure was associated with three potentially life-threatening adverse events.

Another randomized controlled study conducted in Europe also noted no benefit over conventional detoxification without anesthesia on 30-day outcomes (De Jong et al., 2005). Five patients who were detoxified under anesthesia required hospitalization due to adverse events, and the cost of "rapid opioid detoxification" was double that of standard care. In Australia, there is support for detoxification under anesthesia based on the short-term outcomes, but the approach is not cost effective when compared to outpatient procedures (Digiusto et al., 2005; Shanahan et al., 2005).

Protocol for rapid opioid detoxification

The protocol includes pre-anesthetic treatment using adrenergic agents, sedation and insertion of a central line followed by endotracheal intubation. While the patient is under general anesthetic, a nasogastric tube is passed through which a naltrexone slurry is delivered. Patients have to be admitted to an ICU-like setting.

After a number of naltrexone "fill and drain" cycles, with each cycle lasting 45 minutes, the patient is awakened, extubated and sent to recover under usual supervision. The patient is discharged the following morning.

Post-procedural medication includes antiemetics, NSAIDS and supplemental clonidine, as required. The patient is then discharged home with a prescription for oral naltrexone. Some practitioners use naltrexone implants instead because of the advantage they provide in maintaining the patient's abstinence from opioids and the reduced risk of post-detoxification overdose (Hulse, Tait et al., 2005); however, this approach is controversial because there are marked intra- and inter-individual differences in plasma levels (Olsen et al., 2004) and because the implants can cause local tissue complications such as fat necrosis complications (Hamilton et al., 2002; Hulse, Stalenberg et al., 2005).

Patients may be attracted to this form of therapy since it appears to promise a quick fix. It is important for them to understand that "rapid opioid detoxification" has some very significant risks and is not a magic bullet. Moreover, this treatment is expensive, and it has not been demonstrated to be safe for those with comorbid conditions. Therefore, "rapid opioid detoxification" followed by naltrexone implants should be considered an experimental treatment until further study has been completed.

Pharmacological relapse prevention

Naltrexone is theoretically a good option for helping patients to maintain abstinence; however, cost considerations and the low compliance rate with its daily or three-times-per-week dosing reduce its effectiveness. Moreover, most clinicians are concerned about giving naltrexone to patients with hepatitis C, although there is no evidence for increased risk of hepatocellular injury (Brewer & Wong, 2004). Naltrexone implants might, however, become a useful treatment in the future.

Psychosocial counselling

Regardless of the method used to manage the patient's withdrawal, post-withdrawal treatment is always necessary. Patients should begin with an intensive residential or day program, which usually lasts 21 days, followed by aftercare programs that help to maintain abstinence. These programs may be effective for individuals who have strong psychosocial supports, high motivation to avoid relapse and minimal access to opioids. Drug counselling involves addressing external factors and behaviours that lead to drug use and developing alternative healthy behaviours (Woody, 2003).

Psychotherapy, which involves focusing on the resolution of intrapsychic conflict, is not provided in most programs. Most drug counselling and psychotherapy studies have been done on patients who receive methadone; the prognosis for psychosocial treatment in the absence of methadone is poor (Hubbard et al., 2003).

THERAPEUTIC COMMUNITIES

Therapeutic communities are long-term residential facilities that admit patients for 12 months or longer. There appear to be benefits associated with a longer stay, but access to these programs and patient retention are both low. These communities do offer good outcomes for those who stay, however (Keen et al., 2001). Patients who develop a high level of confidence in themselves and have a supportive partner at the time of their discharge are more likely to remain abstinent in the long term (Dekel et al., 2004).

12-STEP TREATMENTS AND AFTERCARE

Attendance at 12-step programs such as NA or AA has been found to be helpful to those who get involved in community service, become a sponsor and develop a network of friends who do not use drugs or alcohol, as well as other supports (Crape et al., 2002; Witbrodt & Kaskutas, 2005). Factors associated with positive attendance include severe levels of dependence and criminality; attachment to a religion does not play a role (Brown et al., 2001). Health care professionals and program staff can facilitate attendance at 12-step programs by keeping an open and positive attitude toward the mutual aid groups and providing factual information about their value (Humphreys, 1999).

Summary

The management of acute opioid withdrawal is necessary but not sufficient for patients to recover from opioid dependence. Abstinence-based treatments should be reserved for carefully selected patients; most patients who meet the criteria for opioid dependence will likely respond better to opioid replacement therapies such as MMT and buprenorphine treatment.

References

Albanese, A.P., Gevirtz, C., Oppenheim, B., Field, J.M., Abels, I. & Eustace J.C. (2000). Outcome and six month follow-up of patients after Ultra Rapid Opiate Detoxification (UROD). *Journal of Addictive Diseases, 19* (2), 11–28.

Amato, L., Davoli, M., Ferri, M., Gowing, L. & Perucci, C.A. (2004). Effectiveness of interventions on opiate withdrawal treatment: An overview of systematic reviews. *Drug and Alcohol Dependence, 73* (3), 219–226.

Brewer, C. & Wong, V.S. (2004). Naltrexone: Report of lack of hepatotoxicity in acute viral hepatitis, with a review of the literature. *Addiction Biology, 9*, 81–87.

Brown, B.S., O'Grady, K.E., Farrell, E.V., Flechner, I.S. & Nurco, D.N. (2001). Factors associated with frequency of 12-step attendance by drug abuse clients. *American Journal of Drug and Alcohol Abuse, 27*, 147–160.

Collins, E.D., Kleber, H.D., Whittington, R.A. & Heitler, N.E. (2005). Anaesthesia-assisted vs. buprenorphine- or clonidine-assisted heroin detoxification and naltrexone induction: A randomized trial. *Journal of the American Medical Association, 294*, 903–913.

Crape, B.L., Latkin, C.A., Laris, A.S. & Knowlton, A.R. (2002). The effects of sponsorship in 12-step treatment of injection drug users. *Drug and Alcohol Dependence, 65*, 291–301.

De Jong, C.A., Laheij, R.J. & Krabbe, P.F. (2005). General anaesthesia does not improve outcome in opioid antagonist detoxification treatment: A randomized controlled trial. *Addiction, 100*, 206–215.

Dekel, R., Benbenishty, R. & Amram, Y. (2004). Therapeutic communities for drug addicts: Prediction of long-term outcomes. *Addictive Behaviors, 29*, 1833–1837.

Digiusto, E., Lintzeris, N., Breen, C., Kimber, J., Mattick, R.P., Bell, J. et al. (2005). Short-term outcomes of five heroin detoxification methods in the Australian NEPOD Project. *Addictive Behaviors, 30*, 443–456.

Hamilton, R.J., Olmedo, R.E., Shah, S., Hung, O.L., Howland, M.A., Peronne, J. et al. (2002). Complications of ultrarapid opioid detoxification with subcutaneous naltrexone pellets. *Academic Emergency Medicine, 9*, 63–68.

Hubbard, R.L., Craddock, S.G. & Anderson, J. (2003). Overview of 5-year followup outcomes in the drug abuse treatment outcome studies (DATOS). *Journal of Substance Abuse Treatment, 25*, 125–134.

Hulse, G.K., Stalenberg, V., McCallum, D., Smit, W., O'Neil, G., Morris, N. et al. (2005). Histological changes over time around the site of sustained release naltrexone-poly (DL-lactide) implants in humans. *Journal of Controlled Release, 108,* 43–55.

Hulse, G.K., Tait, R.J., Comer, S.D., Sullivan, M.A., Jacobs, I.G. & Arnold-Reed, D. (2005). Reducing hospital presentations for opioid overdose in patients treated with sustained release naltrexone implants. *Drug and Alcohol Dependence, 79,* 351–357.

Humphreys, K. (1999). Professional interventions that facilitate 12-step self-help group involvement. *Alcohol Research and Health, 23,* 93–98.

Jasinski, D.R., Johnson, R.E. & Kocher, T.R. (1985). Clonidine in morphine withdrawal. *Archives of General Psychiatry, 42,* 1063–1066.

Keen, J., Oliver, P., Rowse, G. & Mathers, N. (2001). Residential rehabilitation for drug users: A review of 13 months' intake to a therapeutic community. *Family Practice, 18,* 545–548.

Olsen, L., Christophersen, A.S., Frogopsahl, G., Waal, H. & Morland, J. (2004). Plasma concentrations during naltrexone implant treatment of opiate-dependent patients. *British Journal of Clinical Pharmacology, 58,* 219–222.

San, L., Cami, J., Peri, J.M., Mata, R. & Porta, M. (1990). Efficacy of clonidine, guanfacine and methadone in the rapid detoxification of heroin addicts: A controlled clinical trial. *British Journal of Addiction, 85* (1), 141–147.

San, L., Puig, M., Bulbena, A. & Farre, M. (1995). High risk of ultrashort noninvasive opiate detoxification. *American Journal of Psychiatry, 152* (6), 956.

Shanahan, M.D., Doran, C.M., Digiusto, E., Bell, J., Lintzeris, N., White, J. et al. (2005). A cost-effectiveness analysis of heroin detoxification methods in the Australian National Evaluation of Pharmacotherapies for Opioid Dependence (NEPOD). *Addictive Behaviors, 31,* (3), 371-387.

Witbrodt, J. & Kaskutas, L.A. (2005). Does diagnosis matter? Differential effects of 12-step participation and social networks on abstinence. *American Journal of Drug Alcohol Abuse, 31,* 685–707.

Woody, G.E. (2003). Research findings on psychotherapy of addictive disorders. *American Journal on Addictions, 12* (suppl. 2), s19–s26.

SECTION III

Methadone prescribing protocols and guidelines

CHAPTER 7

Methadone dosing guidelines

This chapter discusses general dosing considerations and specific dosing issues for each of the various titration phases, from early stabilization to maintenance.[1]

Overview: Dose and effectiveness

There is good evidence from controlled trials that methadone doses of 60–100 mg are more effective than doses below 60 mg in reducing heroin use and retaining patients in treatment (Goldstein & Judson, 1973). A Cochrane systematic review of 11 randomized, controlled trials and 10 controlled prospective studies concluded that doses at or near 100 mg per day were more effective than lower doses at reducing heroin use and retaining patients in treatment (Faggiano et al., 2003). Another systematic review concluded that doses of 80 to 100 mg are more effective than doses of 60 mg or less (Strain et al., 1999).

There is limited evidence regarding the effectiveness of doses of 120 mg or above compared to doses of 80–100 mg, since few controlled trials have used doses of above 110 mg (Strain et al., 1999; Farre et al., 2002; Faggiano, 2003). One randomized trial found that a fixed dose of 160 mg was no more effective than one of 80 mg, although both were more effective than one of 40 mg (Goldstein & Judson, 1973). In one non-randomized study, patients on an average dose of 211 mg had reduced illicit drug use and improved psychiatric symptoms compared to patients on an average dose of 65 mg (Maxwell & Shindeman, 2002; Maxwell & Shindeman, 1999; Leavitt et al., 2000). There are several reasons for interpreting these results with caution, however: the high-dose group included fewer participants who used injection drugs and more who experienced psychiatric comorbidity, the two groups were based in different clinics, and control patients on doses of 100 to 120 mg seem to have been excluded from some analyses.

SAFETY OF HIGH DOSES

Several case series have demonstrated that patients on very high doses of methadone are at risk for torsades de pointes caused by prolonged QT intervals. In one case series of 17 patients who had experienced torsades, the mean methadone dose was 397 +/– 283 mg and the mean QT interval was 615 +/– 77 msec (Krantz et al., 2002). Many of the patients had other risk factors for arrhythmias (Krantz et al., 2002; Walker et al., 2003; Krantz et al., 2003).

QT prolongation is seen even at lower doses. One study found that patients on a mean methadone dose of 87 mg had QT intervals that were longer than average for their age and gender (Maremmani et al., 2005). A QTC value of greater than 450–460 msec (two standard deviations above the mean) is considered abnormally high, and a value of more than 500 msec is associated with increased mortality (Moss, 1993). Several authors have recommended ECG screening for patients on higher methadone doses or on medications that prolong the QT interval (Maremmani et al., 2005; Vodoz et al., 2003). A recent literature review concluded that patients on doses above 130 mg should have a baseline ECG, and their dose should be reassessed if their QT interval is 470 msec or greater (Krook et al., 2004).

Methadone has been associated with cognitive impairment (level III evidence), although a causal relationship has not been established and the clinical

1 Portions of this chapter were adapted from sections written by the authors for the CPSO *Methadone Maintenance Guidelines*, 2005.

significance of these findings is uncertain. Three studies have demonstrated that patients on methadone maintenance show signs of cognitive impairment as measured by neuropsychological testing, compared to non-drug-using controls (Darke et al., 2000; Mintzer & Stitzer, 2002; Staak et al., 1993). These studies did not control for other factors that might impair cognition, such as previous head injuries and overdoses. Other research has shown that patients generally have significant cognitive impairment shortly after receiving their usual maintenance dose (Curran et al., 2001) and decreased alertness after a large dose increase (Curran et al., 1999). Interestingly, patients in early methadone withdrawal (after 24 hours of abstinence) show greater cognitive impairment and dysphoria than recently dosed patients (Lyvers & Yakimoff, 2003; Dyer et al., 2001).

SERUM LEVELS

There is inconclusive evidence regarding the clinical utility of serum methadone levels. Due to genetic differences in cytochrome P450 activity, the serum levels produced by a given methadone dose vary among individuals, as much as seventeenfold (Eap et al., 2002). Some studies have found an association between low serum methadone levels and drug use (Tennant et al., 1984; Tennant & Shannon, 1995), while others did not confirm this relationship (Bell et al., 1990; Torrens et al., 1998). Similarly, some but not all studies have found an association between withdrawal symptoms and low trough serum levels (Torrens et al., 1998; Borg et al., 1995; Drozdick et al., 2002).

SUMMARY OF DOSING EFFECTIVENESS

Maintenance doses of 60 to 100 mg are more effective than lower doses at reducing heroin use and retaining patients in treatment. The effectiveness of doses above 120 mg has not been established. Methadone use may be associated with cognitive impairment, although the clinical significance of these findings is uncertain and other factors may contribute. Very high methadone doses are associated with torsades de pointes. The clinical utility of serum methadone levels has not been established.

Dose titration and phases

EARLY STABILIZATION PHASE (FIRST TWO WEEKS)

Patients in the first two weeks of methadone treatment are at high risk for death from methadone overdose. In 2000, the mortality rate of patients enrolled in methadone programs in Ontario was 1.7 per 1,000 with most of the deaths occurring in the first two weeks of treatment (Cairns, 2000). This rate is similar to those of other jurisdictions (Caplehorn, 1998; Buster et al., 2002). The risk of fatal methadone overdose for patients during the first two weeks of treatment is estimated to be 98 times higher than that of patients on maintenance doses of methadone, and 6.7 times higher than the risk of a fatal heroin overdose for heroin users not in treatment (Caplehorn & Drummer, 1999).

A death rate of 1.7 per 1,000 is substantially higher than that associated with other common medications. In a review of mortality from NSAIDs, tricyclic antidepressants and phenytoin, only one study reported a mortality rate approaching that of MMT patients—for rheumatoid arthritis patients taking prednisone and NSAIDs without cytoprotection (Fries et al., 1991).

Deaths have been associated with starting doses as low as 30 to 50 mg; a single day's maintenance dose of methadone (50 to 100 mg) can be lethal to non-tolerant adults (Harding-Pink, 1993). In one case series of methadone deaths, the mean methadone dose was 50 mg (Drummer & Opeskin, 1992). In an Australian study (Zador & Sunjic, 2000), the majority of deaths occurred in patients whose physicians had followed the recommended guidelines for initial dosing of 20 to 40 mg of methadone.

The ratio between the maximum recommended initial dose of 30 mg and a potentially fatal single dose of 50 to 70 mg is exceedingly narrow. The comparable ratios for phenytoin, acetaminophen and desipramine are 6:1, 10:1 and 20:1 respectively (Repchinsky, 2003).

Concurrent use of benzodiazepines, alcohol and other sedating drugs substantially increases the risk of methadone overdose death. One study found evidence of polydrug use in 92 per cent of methadone-related deaths (Zador & Sunjic, 2000). Benzodiazepine use causes a fivefold increase in risk of fatal overdose (Caplehorn et al., 2002). In the Ontario coroner's report on methadone overdose deaths, 60 per cent of the deceased patients had benzodiazepines on their toxicology screens, and 30 per cent had alcohol (Cairns, 2000). Animal studies confirm that benzodiazepines increase the lethal effects of methadone (Borron et al., 2002). Other risk factors for methadone toxicity include lack of tolerance, respiratory illness, age, and medications that inhibit methadone metabolism, such as quinolone or macrolide antibiotics, fluconazole and sertraline (Tarumi et al., 2002; Herrlin et al., 2000; Hamilton et al., 2000).

The initial dose

General guidelines

- The recommended initial daily dose is 10 to 30 mg.
- The methadone must be dispensed in a vehicle that does not lend itself to injection.
- The methadone dose must be consumed under the direct supervision of a health professional or an appropriately exempted and trained delegate who is authorized to supervise the ingestion of methadone.

Patients at higher risk for methadone toxicity

Lower doses (10 to 20 mg) should be considered for the following patient groups:

- the elderly and those with underlying respiratory disease
- patients using oral prescription opioids, especially those of low to medium potency such as codeine and oxycodone
- patients using sedating drugs, such as benzodiazepines, alcohol, antipsychotics, sedating antihistamines or other opioids
- patients on drugs that could inhibit methadone metabolism
- patients with lowered opioid tolerance.

Managing high-risk patients

- **Recent benzodiazepine users.** Benzodiazepines are a risk factor for overdose, even if they are being used therapeutically. For patients who have been using high doses of benzodiazepines, it is safer to taper the benzodiazepines before initiating methadone. Consultation with an addiction medicine physician might be considered in this situation. Patients who have been on small doses (e.g., 10 mg diazepam equivalent per day) for many months do not necessarily need to be tapered prior to starting methadone, but they should be started on a lower initial dose.
- **Problem drinkers and alcohol-dependent patients.** Heavy drinkers who are at risk for withdrawal on sudden cessation of alcohol should go through a period of managed withdrawal before methadone initiation. Assistance from an addiction medicine physician is advised. All patients should be advised to abstain from alcohol during early stabilization.
- **Patients who use other sedating drugs.** Patients using antipsychotics and sedating antidepressants are at risk for methadone toxicity, particularly if the sedating drug was recently started, the dose was recently increased, or the dose is moderate or high. A lower initial dose of methadone should be used.
- **Older adults.** Adults over 60 years old with respiratory illness (including chronic illness such as COPD) and acute illnesses such as pneumonia are at risk for methadone toxicity, so lower doses of methadone should be used.
- **Patients who are on drugs that inhibit methadone metabolism.** If the drug is for short-term use only (such as an antibiotic), the physician might recommend that the patient finish the course before prescribing methadone.
- **Patients with lower opioid tolerance.** Lowered opioid tolerance is possible in patients who report non-daily opioid use, daily use of codeine or oral use of prescription opioids at therapeutic doses. A lower initial dose is recommended for this group. Since tolerance is difficult to establish by history, if there is any doubt it is safer to initiate on a lower dose.

Dose adjustment

The dose should be adjusted no more frequently than every three to four days. Dose adjustments are usually in the 5–15 mg range. The size of the increase will depend on the severity of withdrawal and the patient's risk for methadone toxicity.

Clinical criteria for dose increases

The physician should consider increasing the patient's methadone dose if the patient experiences withdrawal symptoms or cravings, or continues opioid use. (Persistent opioid cravings or use may indicate the need for a dose increase, even in the absence of other reported withdrawal symptoms.)

One simple way to assess the adequacy of the dose is to ask the patient how long it "lasts" (i.e., the time interval between taking the methadone and the first appearance of myalgias or other withdrawal symptoms). For example, if the patient takes methadone in the morning and experiences the onset of withdrawal symptoms in the early afternoon, further dosage adjustment is needed. The optimal dose is one that is effective through the night.

Assessment of methadone withdrawal

A patient on inadequate doses of methadone usually describes a characteristic set of symptoms, such as muscle aches, hot flashes, an "electric," restless or uncomfortable feeling, nausea, diarrhea, yawning, fatigue and irritability. The symptoms appear a certain number of hours after the methadone dose, although they may vary to some extent with the patient's activity level and other factors. The onset of symptoms is delayed with each dose increase.

Alternative explanations should be sought if:

- the patient gives an inconsistent history of withdrawal symptoms,
- the patient has one isolated symptom (such as insomnia or nausea),
- the onset of symptoms is not related to the time of the dose, or
- the patient has been on a stable dose and suddenly complains of withdrawal.

It is difficult to completely eliminate mild withdrawal symptoms in the hour or two preceding dosing. A dose might be considered acceptable if the patient sleeps comfortably at night and has only mild withdrawal symptoms on awakening.

Reducing the risk of methadone overdose

The physician should avoid prescribing any sedating drug unless the patient has been on a stable, low dose of the drug for a long period of time. This includes non-benzodiazepine hypnotics, antipsychotics, antidepressants and sedating antihistamines (such as Gravol). Even moderate therapeutic doses of these drugs may increase the risk of overdose if they are initiated at the same time as methadone and the patient is not fully tolerant to their sedating effects.

The physician should carefully review each of the following points with the patient:

- Avoid using all sedating drugs, including alcohol and over-the-counter antihistamines.
- Take the methadone in the morning, since the risk of overdose may be increased at night.
- Do not try to relieve withdrawal symptoms with benzodiazepines, opioids, illicit methadone or other drugs. It takes several weeks to reach the optimal dose of methadone.
- Limit driving or use of machinery after a dose increase, particularly in the first few hours after dosing.
- Store methadone in a locked box. Even single moderate doses can be fatal to both children and adults.
- Do not ever sell or give methadone to an acquaintance, even in small doses. Doing so is dangerous, even if one's intentions are good.
- If several doses are missed, don't take any methadone without consulting with the physician.

Whenever feasible and with the patient's consent, a family member or significant other should be educated about the symptoms of overdose, with clear instructions to go to the emergency department immediately at the first sign of toxicity. Refer to Appendix A of this chapter "Emergency department management of methadone overdose," on page 64.

Additional strategies and precautions for reducing risk

- Educate the patient and his or her family about the risks of other drug use, the risks of non-prescribed methadone use and the signs of methadone toxicity.
- Assess the patient twice a week for the first two weeks.
- Do not prescribe take-home doses ("carries") in the first two months of treatment (see the section "Clinical protocols for take-home doses" on page 77 in Chapter 9).
- If the patient misses one dose in the first two weeks, do not increase the dose for at least two days.
- If the patient misses more than one dose in the first two weeks, titration should be restarted at the initial dose (10–30 mg) for at least three days.

At any stage of methadone treatment, the pharmacy should be instructed to alert the physician if the patient appears sedated or intoxicated. Intoxicated patients should not be medicated until they have been assessed by their physician (see the section "Methadone overdose protocol" on page 60).

Twice-weekly visits are advised during the first two weeks, particularly if the patient is at increased risk for methadone toxicity. If possible, the visits should be scheduled for two to six hours after the methadone dose. The presence of a family member can be helpful. The physician should inquire about sedation and other side-effects.

LATE STABILIZATION PHASE (TWO TO SIX WEEKS)

During the late stabilization phase, a patient usually experiences partial relief from withdrawal symptoms, is only partially tolerant to methadone and often continues to use opioids. As in the early stabilization phase, the dose should be adjusted no more frequently than every three to four days, by 5 to 15 mg. Patients should be seen at least weekly. All dose adjustments require a medical assessment, and the reason for the adjustment should be documented. The prescriber should avoid phone assessments or assessments by non-medical personnel, and should not include automatic dosage adjustments on the prescription.

MAINTENANCE PHASE (SIX WEEKS AND BEYOND)

The maintenance phase usually begins five or six weeks after initiation, by which time a daily dose of 50 to 80 mg has been reached in most cases. Usually, a patient in the maintenance phase has substantially reduced opiate use, is largely tolerant to methadone and experiences minimal or no withdrawal symptoms for most of the day.

Dose increments during the maintenance phase are typically between 5 and 10 mg every five days to two weeks, as necessary. Once a stable dose is established (50 to 120 mg for most patients), the patient should continue to meet with the physician every one to two weeks during the first six to 12 months, depending on the patient's functional stability.

An optimal and stable daily dose will relieve withdrawal symptoms, block opioid-induced euphoria and reduce drug cravings for close to 24 hours, without sedation or other significant side-effects.

Summary dosage adjustment guidelines during late stabilization and maintenance

- Doses should be increased only after the physician has assessed the patient in person and determined that the patient has symptoms of withdrawal or opioid cravings, or is continuing to use opioids.
- During the stabilization phase (two to six weeks), patients should be seen at least weekly, and the dose should be increased by no more than 5 to 15 mg every three or four days.
- During the maintenance phase, or at any time if the dose is 80 mg or more, the dose should be increased by no more than 10 mg every five days to two weeks.

Maintenance doses above 120 mg

Patients on high doses should be granted dose increases if they consistently report a cluster of withdrawal symptoms—including both physical and psychological symptoms—that occur at a predictable time at the end of a dosing interval. The physician should assess the patient for other conditions that are commonly confused with withdrawal (e.g., untreated anxiety disorder, stimulant intoxication, general medical symptoms).

If the patient continues to request additional dose increases despite receiving a dose well above 120 mg, the physician might consider requesting a second opinion from a physician who has experience in addiction medicine and methadone treatment. The opinion should be documented in the chart.

Monitoring peak and trough serum levels might be useful in patients who continue to report withdrawal symptoms despite receiving doses of 120 mg or above (although this approach is controversial because of the subjective nature of withdrawal symptoms and their lack of a clear relationship with serum levels). If the trough level is high, the patient can be reassured that the symptoms are less likely to be caused by withdrawal.

Physicians of patients on high doses should inquire whether the patient or family members have observed cognitive effects that could be attributed to high-dose methadone, such as a tendency to nod off, lethargy and diminished concentration or memory. This is particularly important for patients at risk for cognitive impairment, for example those on sedating drugs.

An ECG is suggested for patients on a methadone dose above 150 mg. The ECG should be repeated for patients on a dose approaching 180 to 200 mg. If the QTc interval is above 470 msec the patient should be referred to a cardiologist, and if it is above 490–500 msec the dose should be carefully tapered. The physician should identify and manage risk factors for arrhythmias (i.e., medications that affect either the QT interval or methadone levels; medications that can trigger arrhythmias, such as cocaine or tricyclic antidepressants; electrolyte abnormalities; or cardiomyopathy).

Prescribers are encouraged to periodically broach the subject of tapering with patients who are on high doses. Clinical experience has found that patients sometimes report feeling more alert and energetic after being tapered from high doses, and some are able to decrease their doses by 20 to 40 mg with relative ease.

A dose should be tapered by no more than 5 mg every one to two weeks. The taper should be held or reversed if the patient reports persistent, uncomfortable withdrawal symptoms.

Summary recommendations for managing patients on doses above 120 mg

- Dosage should be increased only if the patient reports a cluster of withdrawal symptoms toward the end of a dosing interval and/or ongoing opioid use.
- If the patient continues to report withdrawal symptoms despite receiving a high dose, the physician should systematically look for causes of opioid withdrawal and for common conditions that are easily confused with withdrawal.
- A consultation should be considered if the physician has continuing difficulty in stabilizing the patient's dose.
- An electrocardiogram should be obtained for any patient receiving a dose above 150 mg, and repeated for any patient whose dose approaches 180 to 200 mg. Any patient with a QTc interval of 470 msec or above should be referred to a cardiologist, and any patient with an interval of 490–500 msec or above should have the dose reduced. Special caution is required for patients at higher risk for arrhythmias.
- Physicians should periodically attempt a taper for patients on high doses, by no more than 5 mg every one to two weeks. The taper should be held or reversed if the patient reports withdrawal symptoms.

Methadone overdose protocol

Note: The protocol described here is for ambulatory patients; it does not apply to patients who are obtunded or unconscious. Please refer to the protocol on dealing with opioid overdoses in unconscious patients (see Appendix A on page 64).

Patients who may have had an overdose of methadone must be immediately assessed by a physician. During the assessment, the physician should engage the patient in conversation for several minutes and look for early signs of methadone toxicity: sweating, emotional lability, slurred or drawling speech, and nodding off during conversation. Note that patients who have overdosed are often able to remain alert when interacting with others, but succumb to the overdose when they are alone and undisturbed. Therefore, observing the patient's level of alertness while the patient is being quiet is also recommended.

If the additional dose that the patient has received is well above and beyond what would be considered a reasonable dose increase at the particular stage of treatment, the patient should be counselled on the dangers of methadone overdose and advised to go the emergency department.

What constitutes a "reasonable dose increase" depends on the full set of clinical circumstances. For example, if a generally healthy patient has consistently been on 50 mg/d for several weeks and then receives 65 mg by mistake, this would be considered within the range of a reasonable dose increase for that patient. However, if the patient's dose had just been increased to 50 mg the day before and then he or she received 65 mg, this would not be considered a reasonable increase according to the CPSO guidelines. If there is any doubt, the physician (if in Ontario) should call the Ontario Poison Information Centre at 1 800 268-9017.

Clinicians should also keep in mind that even "small" excess doses of methadone can cause toxicity in some circumstances. An extra dose of 15 to 20 mg can cause toxicity during the first two weeks of methadone titration in a patient who is elderly or ill, or in a patient who has taken sedating medication. While fatal overdoses receive the most attention, non-fatal overdoses can have serious consequences, including accidents, aspiration and hypoxic brain damage.

Often the exact amount of methadone a patient has ingested is not known with certainty, so it is best to manage all patients who have taken methadone other than as prescribed as if they have overdosed, even if they report that they are alert and only took "a small amount." The physician should also consider the circumstances under which the methadone was ingested; if it was taken at a party, benzodiazepines or other drugs may have been taken concurrently, increasing the risk of toxicity. Methadone inhibitors can also increase the risk of toxicity. See Chapter 4 for more on methadone pharmacology. A list of drug interactions is available at www.drug-interactions.com.

MANAGEMENT OF SUSPECTED OVERDOSE

In any case of suspected overdose, the patient should be advised on the risks of methadone overdose, including respiratory depression and death. The patient should be given a copy of Appendix A (page 64) and referred to a hospital emergency department. Appendix A should also be faxed to the emergency department, and the physician or responsible person should speak with the attending emergency department physician directly to convey concern and to advise that the patient should be observed for a minimum of 10 hours, and then discharged only if he or she has not displayed any signs of lethargy or sedation during that time.

If the patient refuses to go the emergency department

If the patient refuses to go the emergency department, it is appropriate to fill out a Form 1, which allows an involuntary assessment of the patient. Even if the patient is alert and coherent, he or she has a mental health diagnosis and is also at risk for bodily harm. Opioid-dependent patients' experiences and perceptions can interfere with their ability to make safe decisions. They tend to be far more afraid of withdrawal than they are of overdose, and they know that in the emergency department they may not get methadone and might even be given naloxone. Also, patients and their caregivers may not view signs of methadone toxicity as dangerous—they may consider the signs to be part of the usual state they've experienced countless times before, and assume that they can "handle" it.

If the patient refuses to go to the emergency department and a clinical decision is made to not fill out a Form 1 (e.g., no physician is available on site or the responsible person is speaking to the patient by phone and has not assessed the patient in the preceding week as required by a Form 1), then it is reasonable to send an ambulance or police to the patient's home. In the event that this is absolutely not possible, the patient (and a partner or family member, if available) should be re-instructed on the dangers of overdose and advised to call an ambulance and go to the emergency department at the first sign (such as loud snoring, nodding off or slurred speech).

Emphasize to the patient and any support person with him or her that there is a risk of respiratory depression (slow breathing) and death, and that the greatest risk may be during sleep. Most patients will start to exhibit signs and symptoms of overdose (e.g., sleepiness, sedation) within five hours, although some patients may not exhibit symptoms until 10 hours have passed.

References

Bell, J., Bowron, P., Lewis, J. & Batey, R. (1990). Serum levels of methadone in maintenance clients who persist in illicit drug use. *British Journal of Addiction, 85* (12), 1599–1602.

Borg, L., Ho, A., Peters, J. & Kreek, M.J. (1995). Availability of reliable serum methadone determination for management of symptomatic patients. *Journal of Addictive Diseases, 14* (3), 83–96.

Borron, S.W., Monier, C., Risede, P. & Baud, F.J. (2002). Flunitrazepam variably alters morphine, buprenorphine, and methadone lethality in the rat. *Human and Experimental Toxicology, 21* (11), 599–605.

Buster, M.C., van Brussel, G.H. & van den Brink, W. (2002). An increase in overdose mortality during the first two weeks after entering or re-entering methadone treatment in Amsterdam. *Addiction, 97* (8), 993–1001.

Cairns, J. (2000). *Methadone-Related Deaths in Ontario.* Toronto: Ontario Coroner's Office.

Caplehorn, J.R. (1998). Deaths in the first two weeks of maintenance treatment in NSW in 1994: Identifying cases of iatrogenic methadone toxicity. *Drug and Alcohol Review, 17*, 9–17.

Caplehorn, J.R. & Drummer, O.H. (1999). Mortality associated with New South Wales methadone programs in 1994: Lives lost and saved. *Medical Journal of Australia, 170* (3), 104–109.

Caplehorn, J.R. & Drummer, O.H. (2002). Fatal methadone toxicity: Signs and circumstances, and the role of benzodiazepines. *Australian and New Zealand Journal of Public Health, 26* (4), 358–363.

Curran, H.V., Bolton, J., Wanigaratne, S. & Smyth, C. (1999). Additional methadone increases craving for heroin: A double-blind, placebo-controlled study of chronic opiate users receiving methadone substitution treatment. *Addiction, 94* (5), 665–674.

Curran, H.V., Kleckham, J., Bearn, J., Strang, J. & Wanigaratne, S. (2001). Effects of methadone on cognition, mood and craving in detoxifying opiate addicts: A dose-response study. *Psychopharmacology (Berlin), 154,* (2), 153–160.

Darke, S., Sims, J., McDonald, S. & Wickes, W. (2000). Cognitive impairment among methadone maintenance patients. *Addiction, 95* (5), 687–695.

Drozdick, J. III, Berghella, V., Hill, M. & Kaltenbach, K. (2002). Methadone trough levels in pregnancy. *American Journal of Obstetrics and Gynecology, 187* (5), 1184–1188.

Drummer, O.H. & Opeskin, K. (1992). Methadone toxicity causing death in ten subjects starting on a methadone maintenance program. *American Journal of Forensic Medicine and Pathology, 13* (4), 346–350.

Dyer, K.R., White J.M., Foster, D.J., Bochner, F., Menelaou, A. & Somogyi, A.A. (2001). The relationship between mood state and plasma methadone concentration in maintenance patients. *Journal of Clinical Psychopharmacology, 21* (1), 78–84.

Eap, C.B., Buclin, T. & Baumann, P. (2002). Interindividual variability of the clinical pharmacokinetics of methadone: Implications for the treatment of opioid dependence. *Clinical Pharmacokinetics, 41* (14), 1153–1193.

Faggiano, F., Vigna-Taglianti, F., Versino, E. & Lemma, P. (2003). Methadone maintenance at different dosages for opioid dependence. *Cochrane Database of Systematic Reviews, 3,* CD002208.

Farre, M., Mas, A., Torrens, M., Moreno, V. & Cami, J. (2002). Retention rate and illicit opioid use during methadone maintenance interventions: A meta-analysis. *Drug and Alcohol Dependence, 65* (3), 283–290.

Fries, J.F., Williams, C.A., Bloch, D.A., & Michel, B.A. (1991). Nonsteroidal anti-inflammatory drug-associated gastropathy: Incidence and risk factor models. *American Journal of Medicine, 91* (3), 213–222.

Goldstein, A. & Judson, B.A., (1973). Efficacy and side effects of three widely different methadone doses. *Proceedings. National Conference on Methadone Treatment, 1,* 21–44.

Hamilton, S.P., Nunes, E.V., Janal, M. & Weber, L. (2000). The effect of sertraline on methadone plasma levels in methadone-maintenance patients. *American Journal on Addictions, 9* (1), 63–69.

Harding-Pink, D. (1993). Methadone: One person's maintenance dose is another's poison. *The Lancet, 341* (8846), 665–666.

Herrlin, K., Segerdahl, M., Gustafsson, L. & Kalso, E. (2000). Methadone, ciprofloxacin, and adverse drug reactions. *The Lancet, 356* (9247), 2069–2070.

Krantz, M.J., Kutinsky, I.B, Robertson, A.D. & Mehler, P.S. (2003). Dose-related effects of methadone on QT prolongation in a series of patients with torsade de pointes. *Pharmacotherapy, 23* (6), 802–805.

Krantz, M.J., Lewkowiez, L., Hays, H., Woodroffe, M.A., Robertson, A.D. & Mehler, P.S. (2002). Torsade de pointes associated with very-high-dose methadone. *Annals of Internal Medicine, 137* (6), 501–504.

Krook, A.L., Waal, H. & Hansteen, V. (2004). Routine ECG in methadone-assisted rehabilitation is wrong prioritization. *Tidsskr Nor Laegeforen, 124* (22), 2940–2941.

Leavitt, S.B., Shinderman, M., Maxwell, S., Eap, C.B. & Paris, P. (2000). When "enough" is not enough: New perspectives on optimal methadone maintenance dose. *Mount Sinai Journal of Medicine, 67* (5–6), 404–411.

Lyvers, M. & Yakimoff, M. (2003). Neuropsychological correlates of opioid dependence and withdrawal. *Addictive Behaviors, 28* (3), 605–611.

Maremmani, I., Pacini, M., Cesaroni, C., Lovrecic, M., Perugi, G. & Tagliamonte, A. (2005). QTc interval prolongation in patients on long-term methadone maintenance therapy. *European Addiction Research, 11* (1), 44–49.

Maxwell, S. & Shinderman, M. (1999). Optimizing response to methadone maintenance treatment: Use of higher-dose methadone. *Journal of Psychoactive Drugs, 31* (2), 95–102.

Maxwell, S. & Shinderman, M.S. (2002). Optimizing long-term response to methadone maintenance treatment: A 152-week follow-up using higher-dose methadone. *Journal of Addictive Diseases, 21* (3), 1–12.

Mintzer, M.Z. & Stitzer, M.L. (2002). Cognitive impairment in methadone maintenance patients. *Drug and Alcohol Dependence, 67* (1), 41–51.

Moss, A.J. (1993). Measurement of the QT interval and the risk associated with QTc interval prolongation: A review. *American Journal of Cardiology, 72* (6), 23b–25b.

Repchinsky, C. (Ed.). (2003). *Compendium of Pharmaceuticals and Specialtie 2003: The Canadian Drug Reference for Health Professionals.* Ottawa: Canadian Pharmacists Association.

Staak, M., Berghaus, G., Glazinski, R., Höher, K., Joó, S. & Friedel, B. (1993). Empirical studies of automobile driving fitness of patients treated with methadone-substitution. *Blutalkohol, 30* (6), 321–333.

Strain, E.C., Bigelow, G.E., Liebson, I.A. & Stitzer, M.L. (1999). Moderate- vs high-dose methadone in the treatment of opioid dependence: A randomized trial. *Journal of the American Medical Association, 281* (11), 1000–1005.

Tarumi, Y., Pereira, J. & Watanabe, S. (2002). Methadone and fluconazole: Respiratory depression by drug interaction. *Journal of Pain and Symptom Management, 23* (2), 148–153.

Tennant, F. & Shannon, J. (1995). Cocaine abuse in methadone maintenance patients is associated with low serum methadone concentrations. *Journal of Addictive Diseases, 14* (1), 67–74.

Tennant, F.S., Rawson, R.A., Cohen, A., Tarver, A. & Clabough, D. (1984). Methadone plasma levels and persistent drug abuse in high dose maintenance patients. *NIDA Research Monograph 49*, 262–268.

Torrens, M., Castillo, C., del Moral, E., González, M.L. & de la Torre, R. (1998). Plasma methadone concentrations as an indicator of opioid withdrawal symptoms and heroin use in a methadone maintenance program. *Drug and Alcohol Dependence, 52* (3), 193–200.

Vodoz, J.F., Jaquier, F. & Lamy, O. (2003). Torsade de pointes: A severe and unknown adverse effect in a patient taking methadone. *Schweiz Rundsch Med Prax, 92* (41), 1748–1750.

Walker, P.W., Klein, D. & Kasza, L. (2003). High dose methadone and ventricular arrhythmias: A report of three cases. *Pain, 103* (3), 321–324.

Zador, D. & Sunjic, S. (2000). Deaths in methadone maintenance treatment in New South Wales, Australia 1990–1995. *Addiction, 95* (1), 77–84.

APPENDIX A

Emergency department management of methadone overdose

Patient: ______________________ Physician: ______________________

Relevant details: ____

____

Clinical features: Methadone acts for at least 24 hours, much longer than other opioids. Symptoms begin up to 10 hours after the overdose. Early symptoms include nodding off, drowsiness, slurred speech and emotional lability. Respiratory depression occurs later.

Monitoring: Check frequently for vital signs, respiratory rate and O2 sat, and hold a brief conversation to assess alertness. ECG and cardiac monitoring are recommended to check for prolonged QT interval and ventricular arrhythmias (methadone can cause torsades de pointes).

Recommended time intervals for monitoring suspected overdose:

- Observe for at least 10 hours post-overdose.
- Discharge if patient is completely asymptomatic during that time.
- If patient becomes symptomatic at any time during the 10 hours, observe for at least 24 hours post-overdose.
- If patient is intubated or on naloxone, continue for at least 24 hours post-overdose.
- Monitor for at least six hours after naloxone or intubation is discontinued.

Treatment: Naloxone is a safe treatment in patients who are not physically dependent on opioids (e.g., a patient not in methadone therapy who took methadone at a party). For methadone- or opioid-dependent patients, intubation avoids risks of naloxone-induced withdrawal. Intubation is necessary:

- if RR < 12, hypercapnea is present and desaturation persists despite supplemental oxygen, or
- if the patient fails to respond to naloxone within two minutes.

Recommendations for naloxone dosing:

- If the patient has severe respiratory depression, give 2.0 mg naloxone IV.
- If there is minimal respiratory depression, give 0.01 mg/kg weight to avoid precipitating withdrawal.
- If there is no response after the initial dose, repeat naloxone 2–4 mg every two to three minutes. If there is no response after 10–20 mg naloxone, search for other causes for the coma.
- If the patient responds to naloxone, infuse at two-thirds of the effective dose per hour.
- Give a bolus of one-half the effective dose 15 to 20 minutes after starting infusion.
- Titrate dose to avoid withdrawal, while maintaining adequate non-assisted respirations.

Precautions: Ventricular dysrhythmias and cardiac arrest can occur with naloxone-induced withdrawal, especially if patients are withdrawing from other substances. The patient may become agitated and leave against medical advice (AMA). Watch for naloxone-induced emesis. Intubation avoids these risks.

Departure AMA: If the physician feels the patient is not safe to leave, a Form 1 should be completed and the patient should be forced to stay. Make sure the patient is not in withdrawal.

Discharge: Tell the patient not to take any methadone, alcohol or sedating drugs until seen by a methadone physician the next day. Have a family member or support person observe overnight and call an ambulance if the patient appears more drowsy, is difficult to arouse or snores much more loudly than usual.

CHAPTER 8

Urine drug screening in MMT

This chapter discusses the effectiveness and rationale for drug screens.[1] It explains clinical protocols for urine drug screening, outlines the different laboratory methods used, and lists the urine detection periods for various drugs. The chapter concludes with information on ways to detect and prevent tampering.

Effectiveness of urine drug screens

Urine drug screening (UDS) is the most expensive component of MMT, outweighing the cost of the drug itself and of the physician services. It is thus important to understand the evidence regarding the effectiveness of UDS. The presence of a drug or its metabolite in a biological sample only indicates use or, in some cases, passive exposure. It is never diagnostic of a substance use disorder, which can only be diagnosed clinically.

CONTINGENCY MANAGEMENT

Several controlled trials have demonstrated that contingency management of take-home methadone doses—giving patients "carries" only if their urine is shown to be drug-free—reduces the use of opioids, cocaine and benzodiazepines (Chutuape et al., 1999a, 1999b; Iguchi et al., 1988; Preston et al., 2002; Schmitz et al., 1998; Stitzer et al., 1982). In one randomized trial, 56 per cent of UDS results were negative for those methadone patients who received take-home doses based on a weekly UDS, compared to 10 per cent for those whose carries were determined at random, completely independent of UDS results (Chutuape et al., 2001). Another study showed that contingency management retains its effectiveness in reducing substance use for at least one year after MMT initiation (Preston et al., 2002).

1 Portions of this chapter were adapted from sections written by the authors for the CPSO *Methadone Maintenance Guidelines*, 2005.

UDS VERSUS SELF-REPORTS

Under-reporting of drug use is common; one study found that 60 per cent of cocaine users reported no use although their UDS tests were positive (Myrick et al., 2002). However, when patients report drug use, their UDS results are generally positive (in other words, patients rarely over-report, saying they have been using if they haven't) (Downey et al., 2000). False negative UDS results are also common, and a combination of UDS and self-reports is more accurate than either method used alone. As an example, in one study (Perrone et al., 2001), 57 per cent of patients reported substance use, 62 per cent of UDS samples were positive, and the combination of self-reports and UDS identified substance use in 73 per cent of patients.

FREQUENCY OF TESTING

Evidence suggests that infrequent UDS will fail to detect many cases of substance use, particularly if the use occurs less than daily. There are several reasons for this:

- UDS only detects drugs used over the previous few days
- false negatives are common even within that time period
- patients with some degree of control over their substance use often avoid use prior to the test.

A computer-generated model found that UDS eight times per year (the minimum frequency in methadone programs in the United States) would detect only 50 per cent of daily substance users (Crosby et al., 2003). Twice-weekly testing for cocaine has a higher detection rate than weekly testing (Delucchi et al., 2002); however, the same detection rate can be achieved at half the cost by testing one sample per week, selected at random from two or three samples collected per week (Compton et al., 1996). In a study of 160 patients in four methadone practices, twice-weekly testing detected 50 per cent more illicit opioid use and 70 per cent more cocaine use than less frequent testing (one clinic tested weekly; the other three clinics tested every three to four weeks) (Wasserman et al., 1999).

More frequent testing might also be useful in contingency management of patients who continue to use illicit drugs. In one controlled trial, only 39 per cent of the UDS results were negative for patients receiving carries based on monthly UDS results, compared to 56 per cent for weekly UDS (Chutuape et al., 2001).

There were limitations to the studies cited above: they did not examine the detection rates achieved by combining UDS with patient self-report, and they used subjects who were at an early stage of treatment and/or continued to use illicit drugs. These results cannot be extrapolated to clinically stable patients in long-term treatment whose self-reports and UDS results have consistently been in agreement. Furthermore, there is little evidence that frequent UDS is actually cost-effective in terms of improving outcome. In Ontario, the annual cost per patient of twice-weekly testing approaches $5,000—an enormous cost compared to the other components of MMT. There is concern that frequent testing will reduce patient satisfaction with treatment and therefore decrease treatment retention. Patients identify restrictive practices such as urine drug screening as one reason for their reluctance to engage in methadone treatment (Fischer et al., 2002).

SUMMARY OF EVIDENCE ON UDS

Basing the receipt of take-home doses on successful UDS results has been shown to reduce the use of opioids, cocaine and benzodiazepines. For patients who are in the early stages of treatment or who continue to use drugs, frequent testing has a higher detection rate than infrequent testing and may reduce drug use more effectively. The effects of ongoing frequent UDS on patient outcomes is not known, and further research on the overall effectiveness of UDS is needed.

Clinical protocol for UDS

PURPOSE OF SCREENING

Urine drug screens are used to ensure compliance with methadone treatment and to detect the presence of drugs with abuse potential. UDS is currently the easiest and least intrusive drug-screening method, and can detect use for a longer period before the sample collection than blood-sample methods.

It is important that physicians and other program staff think of UDS as a therapeutic tool for detecting, preventing and managing drug use. Since false positives and negatives are both common, urine drug screens must be interpreted in light of patients' self-reports. In most cases, patients are honest about their drug use if they perceive that their care providers are there to help them and not to "catch" or punish them.

COLLECTION

Sample volume

Although laboratories often require a sample as small as 10 mL, requesting a 40–50 mL sample has advantages: it is more difficult for patients to adulterate or dilute a larger volume or to substitute a large sample for their own, and a minimum of 40 mL is required for temperature testing.

Collection area

The immediate collection area should not have running water, soap, cleaning solutions or other adulterants, especially if patients are not directly supervised. Adding bluing agents or blue food colouring to toilet bowls, urinals and toilet tanks is suggested. Patients who are not directly supervised should be instructed not to flush the toilet until after the sample is surrendered (flushing can create enough noise to cover the transfer of a bogus sample or to collect water for diluting the sample).

Patients should also be discouraged from wearing heavy outer clothing or carrying bags into the collection area.

Baseline UDS

In Ontario, provincial guidelines specify that at least one UDS sample must be collected and interpreted before MMT is initiated. In most cases the baseline sample should be tested using a broad-spectrum (chromatography) test. If the results are inconsistent with the patient's self-report of drug use, the physician may need to re-evaluate the diagnosis of opioid dependence and revise the estimate of the patient's level of opioid tolerance and risk for methadone toxicity. Guidelines for this evaluation are provided in Table 8-1.

In some cases, MMT may be initiated with only a "dipstick" immunoassay, for example when:

- there is unequivocal evidence that the patient is opioid dependent (track marks, documented history of heroin use, etc.)
- the patient is likely to drop out of treatment unless MMT is initiated promptly
- the patient is at high risk for morbidity or mortality if MMT is not initiated promptly (for example, the patient is pregnant, or the patient is homeless and using injection heroin).

Frequency of collection

Most programs test twice per week for at least the first few months (see the discussion above of the cost and benefits of more and less frequent testing). During the early maintenance phase, testing should be continued at least weekly. Ontario guidelines suggest that testing may be decreased to biweekly or monthly after six months of UDS in which the patient consistently tests negative for unauthorized drugs and/or has been given six take-home doses per week.

Physicians must rely on their clinical judgment in establishing individualized testing schedules. Less frequent testing (biweekly or monthly) should be considered for clinically stable patients in the maintenance phase whose UDS and self-reports are consistently negative for drug use. In some circumstances, random biweekly or monthly testing is justified even for patients who use substances—for example, for patients whose self-reports of use have always been consistent with their UDS results, and who do not receive take-home doses.

Physicians should consider increasing the frequency of UDS if the patient:

- has had a slip or relapse,
- is in early recovery from a relapse,
- has become non-adherent,
- has had UDS results that suggest tampering or diversion, or
- has been prescribed a potentially addicting medication.

TABLE 8-1

Interpreting urine drug screen results of MMT patients

CASE	INTERPRETATION
Patient reports daily use of heroin and the UDS is negative for opioids.	The patient may not be opioid dependent.
Patient reports heavy oxycodone use but only codeine is present.	The patient may not be opioid dependent, or may have a low level of opioid tolerance. The patient should be initiated on a lower methadone dose.
UDS is positive for benzodiazepines.	The patient may be at higher risk for methadone toxicity, and should be initiated at a lower methadone dose.

Random testing

Random testing makes it difficult for patients to hide drug use by abstaining for several days prior to the test; however, it is difficult to implement. Random UDS can be organized by assigning a colour, sports team logo or other symbol to each patient. Patients are informed daily by the physician's office of, for example, "today's colour." If that colour matches the patient's, then the patient is required to provide a urine specimen as soon as possible within the next 12 hours. Physicians with a large number of MMT patients will find it easier to have patients call in daily, perhaps on a dedicated phone line with a voice message system. Those with only one or two MMT patients might ask a nurse or receptionist to call patients.

LABORATORY METHODS

Drugs tested for

Drugs routinely tested for using USD include the methadone metabolite EDDP (2-ethylidene-1, 5-dimethyl-3,3-diphenylpyrrolidine), the cocaine metabolite, opioids and benzodiazepines. Other drugs may be tested for depending on individual and regional patterns of substance use.

Testing methods

The two primary types of UDS test are enzyme immunoassay (EIA) and chromatography.

An EIA procedure—for example, EMIT (enzyme multiplied immunoassay technique)—tests for a particular *class* of compound. It uses antibody-antigen reactions to detect compounds that have similar chemical structure, *not necessarily* similar pharmacological properties.

Thus, EIA procedures cannot differentiate between different drugs within the specific group or class. As such, they cannot distinguish morphine from codeine in the opiates group, or amphetamines from methamphetamine—or even from some antihistamines—in the amphetamine group. Nor can opiate assays (which are "tuned" to detect morphine) detect oxycodone or fentanyl, which have different chemical structures but similar pharmacological properties.

All EIA procedures, when performed in a clinical laboratory, have the potential to give quantitative results without any additional costs. Typically, a positive result reflects total concentration of the parent drug(s) plus its metabolite(s) present in the urine.

The trend of urinary concentrations can be a useful guide to assess when lapses occur, to differentiate otherwise abstinent patients from those who have used. For example, continuously elevated values suggest ongoing regular use.

Chromatographic procedures detect individual drug compounds. For example, they differentiate among morphine, codeine, hydromorphone, oxycodone and the metabolite of heroin, monoacetylmorphine.

Chromatography can provide a fairly complete picture of overall drug intake, including the presence of antidepressants, antipsychotics, cardiac drugs, antihistamines and so forth. This profile can assist in monitoring compliance with prescribed drugs other than methadone. It can also help in detecting possible double-doctoring or self-medication.

Each method has its advantages and disadvantages. EIA procedures are less expensive than chromatographic procedures, but they are also more prone to invalidation by adulteration or tampering. They are typically more sensitive, and also more likely to have false positive results. Chromatographic techniques generally have shorter windows of detection than immunoassays, but are more useful for detecting specific drugs.

To ensure accuracy of the results, most methadone practices that use point-of-care immunoassays also send a sample to the lab for chromatography testing at least once per month.

Point-of-care testing

Point-of-care testing uses urine reagent sticks ("dipsticks"), each containing immunoassay tests for several drugs. The most commonly used sticks contain assays for methadone, cocaine, opioids and benzodiazepines. Point-of-care testing has the advantage of giving immediate results; however, it shares the same limitations as other immunoassay methods.

The sensitivity and specificity of the tests can vary depending on the company that produced them. Interpreting the results requires precise timing (the tests must be read a certain number of minutes after they are dipped in the urine). It also involves a measure of subjectivity (determining the presence or absence of a line). Errors usually occur near the detection threshold of the assay.

Detection of different classes of drugs

For a summary of detection times and drug half-lives, see Table 8-2 on page 70.

OPIOIDS

EIA tests can detect opioids for three to five days after last use (but cannot, as explained above, distinguish among specific opioids). Controlled-release opioids can be detected for as long as two weeks. EIA tests often miss semi-synthetic opioids such as oxycodone (although a specific test for oxycodone is now available), and usually miss synthetic opioids such as meperidine and fentanyl. The ingestion of poppy seeds—even of one poppy-seed bagel—will give a positive opiate result (Selavka, 1991). Although this may be considered clinically as a false positive, analytically it is a true positive. (Poppy seeds come from the plant from which morphine is derived.)

Chromatography only detects opioids for one to two days after last use, but it will distinguish between different types of opioids and is more reliable for semi-synthetic and synthetic opioids. Oxycodone and its metabolite, meperidine, fentanyl and norfentanyl are easily detected by chromatographic procedures. Codeine is metabolized to morphine, so both will be detected in a patient on prescribed codeine. The metabolite of heroin, monoacetylmorphine (half-life of 30 min.), is detected by chromatography for a few hours after use.

METHADONE

The EIA test for opioids does not detect methadone, but a specific immunoassay has been developed to screen for it. Compliance is monitored by detection of the methadone metabolite, 2-ethylidene-1, 5-dimethyl-3, 3-diphenylpyrrolidine (EDDP), and of the parent drug. Special-case results:

- If the test is negative for EDDP but positive for the parent compound, this indicates a tampered sample (i.e., a bogus sample that was spiked with methadone).
- If the test is positive for EDDP but negative for the parent compound, the urine pH should first be tested. Methadone is reabsorbed in a basic environment (pH over 7.5). If the urine pH is elevated, the physician should investigate the reason.

BENZODIAZEPINES

EIA techniques will detect diazepam and benzodiazepines that are structurally similar. Because diazepam has a very long half-life and is highly soluble in lipids, it may be detected for up to three weeks after use. Intermediate-acting agents such as lorazepam, bromazepam and, in particular, clonazepam have poor sensitivity and are often undetected.

Chromatography is not used for detecting benzodiazepines.

COCAINE

The cocaine metabolite benzoylecgonine is detected by both EIA and chromatography tests. The parent compound (cocaine) is detected by chromatography for only a few hours after use. New tests do not cross-react with local anesthetics, and inhaling second-hand cocaine smoke will not cause a positive test result.

CANNABIS (THC)

The EIA test for THC is sensitive and specific. THC is sequestered in adipose tissues and released slowly. As a result, it may be detected by USD for a few weeks in chronic users. Occasional users might have positive urine drug tests for several days after the last use.

AMPHETAMINES

Amphetamine EIA tests have a high incidence of false positives due to cross-reactivity with antihistamines and antipsychotics. They need to be combined with chromatography tests to improve specificity and to distinguish between methamphetamine and MDMA (ecstasy).

ALCOHOL

Because alcohol is cleared from the body very rapidly, urine drug screening for alcohol is insensitive, and its cost does not justify its routine use. In one study, case managers of patients with psychiatric disorders identified alcohol use in 32 per cent of the patients, while weekly UDS detected it in only four per cent. Contrast this with the results for other drug use, which managers identified in 45 per cent of the patients, while UDS identified it in 38 per cent (Ries, 2002). In another study of over 200 psychiatric patients in an emergency department, alcohol use in the past three days was detected by history alone in 40 patients and by UDS in only 10 patients (Perrone et al., 2001). The kappa statistic (a measure of concordance between self-report and UDS) was extremely low, only 0.07 (compared to 0.46 for other drugs). Other alcohol screening instruments are more sensitive than UDS. GGT (gamma glutamyl transferase) and the AUDIT screening tool, for example, have sensitivities of 50 to 80 per cent in primary care settings.

TABLE 8-2

Summary of urine detection periods for various drugs

DRUG	HALF-LIFE[2] (T2)	DETECTION PERIOD[3]	COMMENTS
Methamphetamine	12–34 hours	2–3 days	1. If enzyme immunoassay (EIA) is positive, confirmation by chromatography is required because of high incidence of false positives.
Amphetamine (metabolite of methamphetamine)	7–34 hours		2. EIA cross-reacts with phenylpropanolamine, ephedrine, pseudoephedrine, etc.
Methyenedioxy-methamphetamine (MDMA) (ecstasy)	7.6 hours		3. MDMA (ecstasy) and MDA will be detected by the new generation EIA test, but will also cross-react with amphetamine derivatives as in (2).
			4. Chromatography is required to differentiate amphetamine derivatives such as MDA and MDMA.

2 Baselt (2000).
3 The detection period is very much dependent on dose and half-life. The larger the dose, the longer the period that the drug/ metabolite can be detected in the urine.

Continued on next page

TABLE 8-2: SUMMARY OF URINE DETECTION PERIODS FOR VARIOUS DRUGS (continued)

DRUG	HALF-LIFE (T2)	DETECTION PERIOD	COMMENTS
Morphine (metabolite of heroin, codeine, hydromorphone) **Opiates**	1.3–6.7 hours	opiates: 2–4 days (EIA) slow-release opioids: up to 2 weeks	1. EIA does not differentiate between opiates and has a poor sensitivity for oxycodone and meperidine. 2. Even one poppy-seed bagel will be detected on EIA. 3. Chromatography is required in identifying specific opiates (codeine, oxycodone, hydromorphone, hydrocodone, etc.). 4. Chromatography has only a 1–2 day detection period.
Oxycodone	4–6 hours	not detected by opiate EIA test; specific oxycodone assay required	1. Specific oxycodone assay (introduced in 2005) is very sensitive. 2. 33–66% of a single dose is eliminated in 24 hours. 3. Chromatography is required to identify oxycodone and/or its metabolites.
Heroin/ diacetylmorphine (DAM)	60–90 minutes	minutes	DAM is not detected in urine. A positive for opiate (morphine) may indicate heroin use but can also come from use of codeine or morphine.
6-monoacetyl-morphine (MAM)	30 minutes	a few hours	MAM, a specific metabolite of heroin, is detected by chromatography.
Phencyclidine (PCP)	7–16 hours	2–3 days	
Cocaine	30–90 minutes	a few hours	Cocaine is not detected by EIA, but is detected by chromatography.
Benzoylecgonine (metabolite of cocaine)	5–7 hours	3–5 days	Benzoylecgnonine is detected by EIA and chromatography.

Continued on next page

TABLE 8-2: SUMMARY OF URINE DETECTION PERIODS FOR VARIOUS DRUGS (continued)

DRUG	HALF-LIFE (T2)	DETECTION PERIOD	COMMENTS
δ^9-Tetrahydro-cannabinol (THC)	14–38 hours	90% fall in 1 hour (blood)	THC is detected as "cannabinoid" by EIA.
δ^9-Tetrahydro-cannabinoic acid (marijuana metabolite in urine)		a few days to many weeks (depending on chronicity of use)	
Benzodiazepines	a few hours to days	days to weeks (depending on half-life)	1. EIA does not differentiate between different benzodiazepines. Some short-acting agents have poor sensitivity.
Diazepam	15–40 hours	2 weeks or more after last chronic use of diazepam	2. Oxaprozin (Daypro) can cause a false positive.
Flunitrazepam (Rohypnol)[4]	9–25 hours		3. Chromatography is needed to test for the amino derivative of flunitrazepam.
Methadone	15–40 hours ~22–24 hours in chronic patients	1–4 days (in daily users urine should always be positive)	Chromatography or specific EIA is required to distinguish methadone from EDDP.
Barbiturate (phenobarbital)	35–120 hours	1–2 weeks after last use	Chromatography is required to differentiate among various barbiturates.
Alcohol (ethanol)	reduction in blood level by an average of 3.2–3.9 mmol/L/hour or 15–18 mg/100 mL/hour	1.5–12 hours (depending on the peak blood level) (urine typically positive for 1–2 hours after blood alcohol content [BAC] is 0)	1. During the absorption phase urine level lags behind the blood level (i.e., BAC is higher than UAC). 2. During the elimination phase, blood level lags behind urine level (i.e., UAC is higher than BAC).
Gamma-hydroxybutyrate (GHB) ("date rape drug")	0.3–1.0 hour	less than 12 hours	Chromatography is required. Detected as GHB lactone.

4 Flunitrazepam (Rohypnol) is usually not detected with the generic EIA procedure for benzodiazepines. Chromatography should be used to detect amino-flunitrazepam.

Tampering

The prevalence of tampering is not known, but it is probably common. Tampering is usually an attempt to hide a slip or relapse. Patients may be ashamed of the relapse and worry that their physician, therapist or family will be disappointed or angry with them. They may also fear that their right to take-home doses will be taken away if the relapse is discovered.

TAMPERING TECHNIQUES

Substitution

Many ingenious ways have been developed to pass a bogus sample, including the following: strapping plastic bags or condoms to the body with long, small-diameter tubing leading to an artificial penis and the point of voiding; inserting into body cavities small bottles with mouths covered with aluminum foil for easy rupture; and hiding small bottles on the body. Women may wear long full dresses, and men may wear long bulky coats, to help disguise the manipulation of the apparatus at the time of voiding.

Dilution

External dilution involves voiding a small amount of urine and then adding a liquid (water, apple juice, tea, etc.) to increase the volume to the required amount. It can be very effective as a tampering technique, causing the concentration of any drug present to fall below the detection threshold of the assay and give a false negative result.

Waterloading (drinking lots of water to dilute the substance internally) is another common technique and can be very effective. Taking diuretics is also sometimes used in an attempt to affect test results, again with the goal of lowering the concentration of the drug in the urine to a level below the cut-off that the assay can detect, although it is not as effective as dilution.

Adulteration

The intent of this technique, which is usually less effective than substitution or dilution (including waterloading), is to add a substance to a urine specimen to invalidate the test. Ascorbic acid, soap, bleach (powdered or liquid) and salt are among the most commonly used additives.

Raising the alkalinity of one's urine by ingesting sodium bicarbonate or antacids can cause reabsorption of methadone, amphetamines and barbiturates from the urine, making these drugs more difficult to detect. Alkaline urine is of particular interest with patients in an MMT program—at a urine pH of 7.5 or higher, even a daily dose of 100 mg of methadone may produce a negative result due to reabsorption of methadone.

Masking

This technique involves invalidating a drug test by drinking a substance that will mask the drug or alter the test result. Vinegar, the herb goldenseal, zinc sulphate and ASA are examples of substances patients may try to use as maskers. The Internet is replete with products and procedures that claim to assist in producing "clean" urine. Most attempts at masking are ineffective.

METHODS FOR DETECTING AND PREVENTING TAMPERING

Preventing dilution

Using bluing agents in toilets is recommended. Running water should not be available in the area where patients produce samples.

Testing for methadone metabolite

EDDP should be routinely tested for in order to detect substituted samples to which methadone has been added. Both EIA and chromatography methods are now available.

Direct observation

Observation may deter patients from tampering with their samples.

Temperature testing

If a patient is unable to void while under direct observation, or if attendants are not available for supervision, temperature testing can be useful for detecting substituted samples. Patients may try to keep samples warm through insulating the container, keeping them close to the body, or heating them with heating pads worn on the body or with hot water in the bathroom, but these measures usually fail to keep the sample at body temperature.

Temperature testing must be done immediately after the sample is provided because urine temperature falls rapidly. Test the temperature with a rapid-response electronic thermometer or a temperature strip; regular alcohol or mercury thermometers do not respond quickly enough. A minimum sample size of 40 mL is needed to avoid excessive ambient cooling. The normal temperature range of a urine sample is 34°C–36°C within one minute of voiding, and 32°C–36°C within four minutes.

Measuring creatinine

Creatinine is a better marker of dilution than specific gravity. Abnormally low creatinine levels (below 2 or 3 mg/dL) suggest dilution or waterloading. Age and gender are factors in urine creatinine levels.

Measuring sodium chloride

Normal ranges are 20–230 mmol/L for sodium, and 15–250 mmol/L for chloride. Elevated urine sodium (>280 mmol/L) and chloride (>280 mmol/L) could indicate the presence of adulterants such as bleach or table salt.

Measuring urine pH

The normal range is 5.5–7.5. A urine pH of less than 5.0 or greater than 8.0 suggests adulteration, although urinary tract infections and certain diets can also elevate pH. Tea-coloured "Urine Luck," an additive used to adulterate samples, will cause the urine pH to fall below 4.0.

"Fingerprinting"

Two patients may attempt to submit the same "clean" urine sample, or one patient may attempt to submit the same sample on two different occasions. This should be suspected if each of the four analytes—urine pH, sodium, chloride and creatinine—of two samples are within two or three per cent of each other (Kapur et al., 1999).

MANAGEMENT OF COMMON PROBLEMS IN URINE DRUG SCREENING

Patient can't void while observed

If the patient is unstable or thought to be at risk for tampering, weekly or twice-weekly UDS plus temperature testing is suggested as an alternative. For stable patients, unsupervised UDS may be acceptable.

Patient suspected of tampering

There is little empirical evidence on the prevalence, causes or prevention of tampering. Many experienced clinicians are of the opinion that tampering might be reduced if patients understand the therapeutic rationale for program rules, if program policies are flexible and not viewed as punitive, and if patients have a strong therapeutic alliance with their physicians or therapists.

If tampering is suspected, whenever possible a second sample should be obtained immediately. Program staff may wish to obtain and carefully analyze several samples over the next few weeks before confronting the patient. If three consecutive samples have low creatinine or abnormal temperature ranges, then lab error or biological variation is less likely.

If the patient acknowledges tampering to hide a relapse, the usual strategies for managing relapse should be implemented. The patient should be advised on more positive ways to deal with relapse. The physician should emphasize that tampering is a serious breach of the treatment agreement and may lead to consequences, such as prolonged loss of take-home dose privileges.

Patients who continue to deny tampering despite strong evidence should be managed as if they had relapsed. They should be monitored very carefully with UDS to look for evidence of continued drug use or tampering.

Patient does not adhere to the collection schedule

This can be a major problem for methadone providers whose patients attend community pharmacies and laboratories. Patients sometimes feel that UDS is humiliating, time-consuming and unnecessary if they have been honest with their physician about their substance use. They may make excuses for why they have not provided samples, or they may insist that they have done so but that the laboratory failed to send the report to the physician.

In these circumstances, UDS collection can be facilitated by having the laboratory technician initial and date a card or chit at the time a sample is collected, and then requiring the patient to show this card to the pharmacist before the methadone is dispensed. Alternatively, the physician might time the methadone prescription to end on the expected UDS collection date, and ensure that his or her office does not give or fax a new prescription until the patient supplies proof that a sample has been left.

If a patient continues to disregard the collection schedule, the physician should reassess his or her take-home dose privileges.

UDS is positive but patient denies use

The physician should explore possible explanations, particularly if the patient's self-reports have generally been consistent with his or her UDS results.

- *False positives* should be ruled out (e.g., poppy seeds for opioids, antihistamines for amphetamines). Since false positives are more common with EIA techniques, any positive result obtained this way should be confirmed using chromatography.
- *Inadvertent drug use* should be considered. Patients should be advised not to take any medication from a friend or relative, even if they are assured that it is harmless. Patients who claim that their cannabis was laced with cocaine should be advised that they must stop cannabis use or ensure a "safer" supply. A first episode of inadvertent drug use may be managed through patient education, but ongoing positive tests resulting from such use should be managed as relapses.
- *Relapse* should be considered. If the patient continues to deny use despite a confirmed positive UDS result, the physician should manage the situation as a relapse, using frequent testing (as often as twice per week).

UDS is negative for a prescribed medication

Both EIA and chromatography tests can have false negatives (the likelihood depends on the amount of drug taken, the amount of water consumed and various pharmacokinetic and renal factors). The physician should take a careful history of drug use in the days prior to the test.

If the prescribed drug is sold on the street (e.g., oxycodone) and chromatography tests for it are consistently negative, diversion should be suspected. Weekly or twice-weekly monitoring might be necessary for a few weeks to confirm this suspicion. If it is confirmed, the patient must be confronted and his or her take-home dose privileges should be reassessed.

Patient faces serious consequences for even one positive sample

In such circumstances (for example, the patient is on parole or under the supervision of Children's Aid), the physician should pre-arrange with the lab for confirmatory testing. The lab must keep the sample for at least two weeks, report positive results to the physician immediately, and retest all positive samples using a different method. At present, gas chromotography–mass spectrometry (GC-MS) is the gold standard for confirmatory testing.

References

Baselt, R.C. (2000). *Disposition of Toxic Drugs and Chemicals in Man* (5th ed.) Foster City, CA: Chemical Toxicology Institute.

Chutuape, M.A., Silverman, K. & Stitzer, M. (1999a). Contingent reinforcement sustains post-detoxification abstinence from multiple drugs: A preliminary study with methadone patients. *Drug and Alcohol Dependence, 54* (1), 69–81.

Chutuape, M.A., Silverman, K. & Stitzer, M.L. (1999b). Use of methadone take-home contingencies with persistent opiate and cocaine abusers. *Journal of Substance Abuse Treatment, 16* (1), 23–30.

Chutuape, M.A., Silverman, K. & Stitzer, M.L. (2001). Effects of urine testing frequency on outcome in a methadone take-home contingency program. *Drug and Alcohol Dependence, 62* (1), 69–76.

Compton, P.A., Ling, W., Wesson, D.R., Charuvastra, V.C. & Wilkins, J. (1996). Urine toxicology as an outcome measure in drug abuse clinical trials: Must every sample be analyzed? *Journal of Addictive Diseases, 15* (2), 85–92.

Crosby, R.D., Carlson, G.A. & Specker, S.M. (2003). Simulation of drug use and urine screening patterns. *Journal of Addictive Diseases, 22* (3), 89–98.

Delucchi, K.L., Batki, S.L., Moon, J., Jacob, P. III & Jones, R.T. (2002). Urine toxicology samples in cocaine treatment trials: How many need to be tested? *Journal of Addictive Diseases, 21* (2), 17–26.

Downey, K.K., Helmus, T.C. & Schuster, C.R. (2000). Contingency management for accurate predictions of urinalysis test results and lack of correspondence with self-reported drug use among polydrug abusers. *Psychology of Addictive Behaviors, 14* (1), 69–72.

Fischer, B., Chin, A.T., Kuo, I., Kirst, M. & Vlahov, D. (2002). Canadian illicit opiate users' views on methadone and other opiate prescription treatment: An exploratory qualitative study. *Substance Use and Misuse, 37* (4), 495–522.

Iguchi, M.Y., Stitzer, M.L., Bigelow, G.E. & Liebson, I.A. (1988). Contingency management in methadone maintenance: Effects of reinforcing and aversive consequences on illicit polydrug use. *Drug and Alcohol Dependence, 22* (1–2), 1–7.

Kapur, B., Hershkop, S., Koren, G. & Gaughan,V. (1999). Urine fingerprinting: Detection of sample tampering in an opiate dependency program. *Therapeutic Drug Monitoring, 21* (2), 243–250.

Myrick, H., Henderson, S., Dansky, B., Pelic, C. & Brady, K.T. (2002). Clinical characteristics of under-reporters on urine drug screens in a cocaine treatment study. *American Journal on Addictions, 11* (4), 255–261.

Perrone, J., De Roos, F., Jayaraman, S. & Hollander, J. (2001). Drug screening versus history in detection of substance use in ED psychiatric patients. *American Journal of Emergency Medicine, 19* (1), 49-51.

Preston, K.L., Umbricht, A. & Epstein, D.H. (2002). Abstinence reinforcement maintenance contingency and one-year follow-up. *Drug and Alcohol Dependence, 67* (2), 125–137.

Ries, R.K., Dyck, D.G., Short, R., Srebnik, D., Snowden, M. & Comtois, K.A. (2002). Use of case manager ratings and weekly urine toxicology tests among outpatients with dual diagnoses. *Psychiatric Services, 53* (6), 764-766.

Schmitz, J.M., Rhoades, H.M., Elk, R., Creson, D., Hussein, I. & Grabowski, J. (1998). Medication take-home doses and contingency management. *Experimental and Clinical Psychopharmacology, 6* (2), 162–168.

Selavka, Carl M. (1991). Poppy seed ingestion as a contributing factor to opiate-positive urinalysis result: The Pacific perspective. *Journal of Forensic Sciences, 36*, 685–696.

Stitzer, M.L., Bigelow, G.E., Liebsob, A. & Hawthorne, J.W. (1982, 1992). Contingent reinforcement for benzodiazepine-free urines: Evaluation of a drug abuse treatment intervention. *Journal of Applied Behavior Analysis, 15* (4), 493–503.

Wasserman, D.A., Korcha, R., Havassy, B.E. & Hall, S.M. (1999). Detection of illicit opioid and cocaine use in methadone maintenance treatment. *American Journal of Drug and Alcohol Abuse, 25* (3), 561–571.

CHAPTER 9

Take-home doses

This chapter discusses the effectiveness and safety of take-home doses, as well as the clinical protocols used to manage them, such as patient agreements.[1]

Effectiveness and safety of take-home doses

Controlled trials have demonstrated that granting patients take-home dose privileges if their urine screens are drug-free is effective in reducing substance use. Surveys and observational studies suggest that patients strongly value being able to take home doses (Amass et al., 1996), and treatment retention rates are lower in clinics with restrictive take-home policies. In 1972 a large methadone program in Boston instituted a no-take-home policy, and its dropout rate increased fivefold—after 10 months only 43 per cent of patients remained in treatment. Other studies have had similar results (Pani et al., 1996).

Unfortunately, diversion of prescribed methadone is common (Fountain et al., 2000). There is a large street market for methadone, which sells for between 50 cents and one dollar per milligram. Diversion is the major cause of methadone overdose deaths. Between 1996 and 2000 in Ontario, 151 of 194 methadone-related deaths were attributed to diverted methadone (Cairns, 2000). Studies in other jurisdictions have had similar results (Vormfelde & Poser, 2001).

While banning take-home doses would reduce methadone diversion, it could have an adverse impact overall. It would almost certainly cause a substantial number of opioid-dependent patients to drop out of MMT, or dissuade them from enrolling in the first place. Only 15 to 20 per cent of opioid-dependent patients are on methadone treatment in Canada, and potential clients cite restrictive policies as a barrier to entering and staying in treatment (Fischer et al., 2002). People who drop out of treatment face a substantially higher risk of mortality than patients in MMT. Thus, while restrictive take-home policies can reduce mortality from diversion, they may increase total mortality by increasing the population of untreated opioid users. Further research is needed in this area.

Clinical protocols for take-home doses

The decision to prescribe take-home doses is based on three considerations: the patient's clinical stability, contingency management and the risk of diversion.

CLINICAL STABILITY

A physician should allow take-home doses only when the patient demonstrates the ability to store and use the methadone safely and responsibly. To establish whether this is the case, the following factors should be considered:

- Does the patient have a medical or psychiatric condition that affects his or her ability to use take-home doses safely? Take-home doses might pose a risk in patients with suicidal ideation, active psychosis, encephalopathy or dementia.
- Is the patient able to safely store the methadone in a locked box? Since methadone can be fatal when consumed by non-tolerant individuals, patients must be able to store it safely. This can be difficult for patients who are homeless or in temporary housing. Some programs require that patients show the pharmacist or physician their locked box.

1 Portions of this chapter were adapted from sections written by the authors for the CPSO *Methadone Maintenance Guidelines*, 2005.

- Is the patient on a stable methadone dose? Patients in early titration might use their take-home doses to relieve withdrawal symptoms. In Ontario, no take-home doses are allowed in the first two months of treatment.
- Is the patient currently abusing drugs? Patients who are actively abusing or dependent on alcohol, benzodiazepines, cocaine or other drugs can misuse take-home doses in several ways. They may sell their doses to purchase drugs, they may increase their drug use to relieve withdrawal symptoms or dysphoria, or they may put themselves at risk for overdose by combining their methadone with other drugs.
- Is the patient compliant with the treatment program? Non-compliance can indicate clinical instability. Patients who regularly miss clinic appointments, scheduled UDS collections or required pharmacy attendance should have their take-home status reviewed.

CONTINGENCY MANAGEMENT

Take-home dose privileges are highly valued by methadone patients and are a powerful incentive for behavioural change. Most programs use a modified contingency management approach, granting take-home doses gradually to patients whose urine drug screens and self-reports confirm no problematic drug use. In Ontario, one take-home dose per week is allowed in the third month of treatment, two doses per week in the fourth month, and so on. (See Table 9-1)

A physician may decide not to reduce the level of a patient's take-home dose privileges following a single episode of drug use, if the episode has resolved and if the patient remains clinically stable. To help prevent a relapse, the physician should consider increasing the frequency of office visits, urine drug screens and counselling support.

During a sustained relapse, it is usually safest to discontinue all take-home doses. Using a contingency management approach, the physician may then prescribe one new take-home dose per week for each negative urine sample. Thus, a patient who had been taking home six doses per week (the maximum possible) would need to have six consecutive negative UDS results over six or more weeks before the full privileges were reinstated.

TABLE 9–1

Take-home dose schedule

CRITERIA: THE PATIENT IS CLINICALLY STABLE, HAS NO PROBLEMATIC DRUG USE AND HAS . . .	NUMBER OF TAKE-HOME DOSES PER WEEK
been on methadone for at least two months	1
received one take-home dose per week for at least one month	2
received two take-home doses per week for at least one month	3
received three take-home doses per week for at least one month	4
received four take-home doses per week for at least one month	5
received five take-home doses per week for at least one month	6

RISK OF DIVERSION

Diversion of prescription methadone can lead to serious results, including death. For reasons of public safety, patients who are strongly suspected of diverting their methadone should not be given take-home doses. If a patient is routinely selling substantial portions of his or her daily methadone dose, the dose should be reduced to avoid exposing him or her to toxicity (see Chapter 7, "Methadone dosing guidelines").

A patient's take-home doses should only be reintroduced if the physician is confident that the patient will no longer attempt to sell the methadone. For example, if the patient was diverting because of a sustained relapse to cocaine, but has attended a treatment program and has been abstinent for over six months, a gradual reintroduction of take-home dose privileges may be considered, with an agreement that they will be rescinded if the patient relapses.

Diversion should be suspected in patients who are found to tamper with their urine (see the section "Tampering" on page 73 in Chapter 8), although relapse is also a common reason for urine tampering. Accusations by fellow patients are *not* grounds for rescinding take-home dose privileges unless the physician is convinced the accusers are credible. Greater confidence should be placed in reports from patients who don't know the patient suspected of diversion, reports from multiple sources, staff witnesses to conversations about diversion, or concrete evidence (e.g., someone brings in an empty methadone bottle labelled with the patient's name).

If there is reason to suspect diversion, "callbacks" can be used to determine if the patient is adherent: the patient is instructed to return, within 24 hours, the remaining doses for the week. The returned bottles are then analyzed for methadone content. If a bottle's dose is significantly lower than predicted, the patient is either taking extra methadone or diverting it. (The latter is particularly likely if the patient is on a high dose and/or repeatedly requests dose increases.) In either case, the take-home doses should be cancelled for safety reasons.

NON-PROBLEMATIC SUBSTANCE USE

A patient may receive take-home doses even if a UDS indicates the presence of a potentially addicting substance, if:

- the use is occasional and there is no evidence of harm (e.g., weekend cannabis use), or
- the patient is taking the substance as prescribed by a physician (e.g., benzodiazepines for anxiety).

Physicians need to use their judgment to distinguish non-problematic use from abuse or dependence. Non-problematic use of cannabis is much more common than non-problematic use of cocaine or heroin, but cannabis use can be a problem. For example, a patient who smokes four cannabis joints a night might well be dependent on it, indicating that the take-home status and treatment plan should be reviewed.

Patient education and special issues

Physicians should advise patients of the risks of take-home doses, and make clear that patients must store their methadone in locked containers. Where practical, a spouse or significant other should be present for the initial discussion on take-home dosing.

THE TAKE-HOME AGREEMENT

A written take-home agreement ("carry agreement") can facilitate communication. This document, which the patient signs, is kept as part of his or her chart. It should include information on the risks of methadone use by children or non-tolerant adults, and it should stress the need for safe storage of medication. It should also emphasize the importance of adhering to the schedule of clinic appointments and attendance at the pharmacy. The agreement should state that the physician may at any time initiate a callback, which requires the patient to present the bottles for all take-home doses for that week, both used and unused. (Such a callback should take place only when there is an established protocol to analyze the contents of the bottles and the physician is confident that there has been no error in the preparation of the methadone in the pharmacy.)

USE OF MEDICATIONS WITH ABUSE POTENTIAL

MMT patients who are prescribed opioids, benzodiazepines or other potentially addicting drugs may receive more than one take-home dose per week if they have a medical diagnosis that warrants the use of the medication, such as severe generalized anxiety disorder for which benzodiazepines have been prescribed, attention-deficit/hyperactivity disorder (ADHD) being treated with methylphenidate or chronic pain being managed with opioids.

However, physicians should keep in mind that these medications make it difficult to interpret urine drug screens and may place the patient at higher risk for abuse and dependence. Certain precautions should be observed:

- The prescriber should ensure that the patient meets clinical criteria for the medical or psychiatric condition in question and has received an adequate trial of non-addicting therapies.
- The patient should not be prescribed any medication that he or she has been addicted to in the past.
- Where possible, drugs with a lower abuse liability (e.g., oxazepam) are preferred over drugs with a higher liability (e.g., diazepam).
- The medication should be prescribed at the lowest effective dose.
- An addiction medicine specialist should be consulted if the prescriber has any concerns about the appropriateness of the medication.

If the patient's family physician is prescribing the medication, he or she should be aware of the patient's past addiction history and of all currently prescribed medications, and the patient must provide consent for free communication between the family physician and the methadone prescriber.

TEMPORARY TAKE-HOME PRIVILEGES

Medical disability

If a patient is medically unable to visit the pharmacy, a physician may temporarily prescribe take-home doses to be supervised by a relative, although such exceptions should be viewed as temporary and subject to frequent reassessment.

The physician should be confident that the relative understands his or her responsibility to dispense the methadone as prescribed, and should keep in mind that such supervision may nevertheless not be as safe as that provided by a health professional. Once the disability resolves, the usual take-home schedule should be resumed.

If a patient is receiving opioids, benzodiazepines or other psychoactive medications for the medical condition, these could interact with the methadone or put the patient at risk for relapse. In these circumstances, the physician must carefully decide whether the benefits of prescribing take-home doses outweigh the risk of further destabilizing the patient.

Compassionate grounds

MMT patients may be provided short-term take-home doses on a compassionate basis in cases of personal or family crises. Before granting such an exception, the physician should verify the extenuating circumstances and be satisfied that there is no other way to have the patient's dosing observed (e.g., at a local pharmacy). In addition, the physician should be satisfied that the patient is clinically stable and able to store and handle take-home doses safely.

Travel for job or vacation

MMT patients who meet criteria for a high level of take-home privileges (i.e., only one or two observed doses per week) may be temporarily granted a higher number of carries in order to travel for a vacation or work. The Ontario guidelines support take-home dose extensions of up to 14 days for this purpose. The particular reason for the extension should be documented, and the patient should provide the physician with verification of the travel plan (e.g., a plane ticket or letter from work).

It may also be possible for the patient to receive supervised doses at his or her destination. Many MMT programs in North America and Europe will provide "courtesy dosing": they will dispense methadone at the travelling patient's usual dose and take-home schedule. To arrange this, the physician must send the program a letter confirming the patient's identity and dose, and the intended duration of the stay. Physicians can contact the CPSO Methadone Program for information about available programs.

Lost take-home doses

MMT patients whose take-home medication is lost or stolen are usually expected to report the loss to the police and to attend the pharmacy daily for supervised dosing for the duration of the period affected. In case of such a loss, the physician should reassess the patient's clinical stability, and may choose to reduce the level of take-home dose privileges.

References

Amass, L., Bickel, W.K., Crean, J.P., Higgins, S.T. & Badger, G.J. (1996). Preferences for clinic privileges, retail items and social activities in an outpatient buprenorphine treatment program. *Journal of Substance Abuse Treatment, 13* (1), 43-49.

Cairns, J. (2000). *Methadone-Related Deaths in Ontario.* Toronto: Ontario Coroner's Office.

Fischer, B., Chin, A.T., Kuo, I., Kirst, M. & Vlahov, D. (2002). Canadian illicit opiate users' views on methadone and other opiate prescription treatment: An exploratory qualitative study. *Substance Use and Misuse, 37* (4), 495–522.

Fountain, J., Strang, J., Gossop, M., Farrell, M. & Griffiths, P. (2000). Diversion of prescribed drugs by drug users in treatment: Analysis of the U.K. market and new data from London. *Addiction, 95* (3) 393–406.

Pani, P.P., Pirastu, R., Ricci, A. & Gessa, G.L. (1996). Prohibition of take-home dosages: Negative consequences on methadone maintenance treatment. *Drug and Alcohol Dependence, 41* (1), 81–84.

Vormfelde, S.V. & Poser, W. (2001). Death attributed to methadone. *Pharmacopsychiatry, 34* (6), 217-222.

CHAPTER 10

Termination of MMT

This chapter begins with a discussion of voluntary and involuntary termination of MMT, including safe discharge and transfer of care. It also describes patient indicators for successfully ending treatment, symptoms associated with this phase of treatment and guidelines for successfully tapering doses.

Ending the doctor-patient relationship

Terminating a patient's MMT may also mean terminating the therapeutic relationship. This disengagement can be a complex issue and needs careful planning in order to be managed effectively (Stokes et al., 2004). The patient should understand the risks and benefits of withdrawing from MMT.

The patient, the physician or both may decide to end the relationship (Hayes-Bautista, 1976). Ideally, discharge should be a voluntary process, although in some circumstances, involuntary discharge from care is necessary, such as when there are threats of violence against staff or other patients. Regardless of the reason for discharge, a physician is legally and ethically bound to continue treating a patient until that patient:

- no longer requires or wants the doctor's services,
- is transferred to another suitable physician or treatment program, or
- receives adequate notice that the doctor intends to end the therapeutic relationship.

VOLUNTARY TERMINATION OF MMT

When a patient wishes to discontinue methadone treatment voluntarily, the physician needs to explore several factors, such as the prognosis for dose tapering, the best process and pace for tapering, and the appropriate follow-up once the taper is complete.

Patient prognosis with termination of MMT

The relapse rates for patients who leave MMT are high (Dole & Nyswander, 1976). Those who terminate treatment have a higher risk of death and increased alcohol use (Eklund et al., 1995). More than 50 per cent of those who attempt to terminate are unable to do so. However, those who are successful—those who taper off their methadone dose to completion—report an improvement in their quality of life. Not surprisingly, the prognosis is best for those who leave voluntarily because they have done well in MMT: 46 per cent of such subjects in one study remained abstinent after an average of 2.5 years after their MMT had ended, whereas patients who drop out of MMT or are discharged from their programs for non-adherence have a seven per cent rate of abstinence (Cushman, 1978).

Observational studies suggest that the outcome of tapering off methadone use is likely to be better for patients who have been in MMT for two to three years or longer than for patients who have spent less than two years in MMT (Stimmel et al., 1978; Cushman, 1981).

Data from the United States demonstrate that those who stayed in treatment for only six to 12 months were more likely to be using heroin at a five-year follow-up than those who stayed in treatment for a year or longer (Hubbard et al., 2003).

Pace of methadone tapering

Methadone should only be stopped abruptly in cases of acute overdose or allergic reaction. Abrupt termination of methadone may precipitate acute withdrawal, which is characterized by autonomic dysfunction, craving and restlessness. The onset is usually gradual (e.g., over a period of 12 to 48 hours) and peaks three to four days after the last dose is taken. It can last for 15 to 20 days. Subacute withdrawal symptoms can persist for months; however, most patients relapse to other opioid use or resume methadone treatment before withdrawal becomes unmanageable.

Slow tapering is more successful than rapid tapering (Senay et al., 1977). In the case of a voluntary taper, it is recommended that the daily dose not be decreased by more than 10 per cent of the dose every five to seven days. Using a percentage rather than a fixed amount (e.g., 5 mg per week) as a guide to the size of the reduction is recommended, since tapering by a fixed amount may precipitate withdrawal as the total daily dose falls below 20 mg per day. Peak dysphoric symptoms generally occur at doses of 5 to 10 mg per day (Kanof et al., 1993).

In clinical practice, tapering as slowly as 1 to 2 mg every one to two weeks has been successful. The pace of tapering should in part be guided by the patient's ability to tolerate the process. It should be halted or reversed at the patient's request if he or she complains of cravings, withdrawal or relapse. Sudden, unexpected stressors, such as the loss of a job, a divorce or other break-up, or loss of custody of a child, may also be reasons to halt the tapering process until the patient's response to the stressor is assessed and found to be satisfactory.

Boundary setting

It is important for physicians to set appropriate boundaries so that patients can disengage from treatment effectively. Some patients may feel extreme gratitude toward their physicians; some may come to feel dependent; and for some, the ongoing treatment process may have provided an important healthy, supportive relationship, which they may fear losing. In such cases, patients may make unnecessary appointments that have little therapeutic benefit but are simply social visits. If the physician identifies a fear of disengagement, it is important to explore these fears with the patient and help resolve them. Physicians must also continue to follow the rules of the CPSO in maintaining appropriate boundaries with ex-patients once their treatment is complete.

PATIENT DISCONTINUANCE AGAINST MEDICAL ADVICE

Some patients, in spite of a demonstrated or potential benefit from methadone, elect to discontinue MMT. The risk of such discontinuation is usually highest in the first few months of treatment, possibly due to psychosocial factors, clinical factors and unmet expectations of treatment. Patients who make this decision should be offered help in exploring it. It is important for physicians to understand the process of change and be available if the patient wishes to re-engage in therapy.

INVOLUNTARY DISCHARGE

Various factors can lead a physician to decide to terminate the therapeutic relationship with a patient. If it is not possible to safely transfer the care of the patient to another prescriber, the physician still has the right to discontinue treatment. However, it is contraindicated to involuntarily taper a patient's methadone treatment due to ongoing drug use or failure to attend therapy sessions as part of a contingency management program.

The decision to discharge the patient may need to be precipitous if there have been threats to staff or other patients in the practice and disruptive or violent behaviour by the patient.

SAFE AND EFFECTIVE DISCHARGE

Notwithstanding the reasons for the discharge, the process is important. All rules that govern the termination of a doctor-patient relationship apply.

When a patient is to be discharged from an MMT program, the reasons for discharge, the timeline and the process to be followed should be communicated clearly to the patient and well documented. The timeline should provide the patient a reasonable amount of time to find another prescriber—how much time is reasonable will vary according to the location and the available resources. The patient could be referred to the CPSO for help in finding another physician. The documentation of the discharge should include a letter to the patient giving official notice of terminating the relationship, a copy of which should be kept on file. To make sure the patient receives it, this notice could be sent via registered mail with an acknowledgment due upon receipt.

MMT patients who are being discharged involuntarily and who cannot be transferred to another treatment setting should have their doses tapered slowly—by no more than 10 per cent every three to four days. Clonidine may be used in the final one to two weeks of the taper, as it shortens the duration of withdrawal symptoms (Milby, 1988)—the recommended dose is 0.1 mg po tid–qid for five to seven days. However, at least once per week blood pressure monitoring is recommended for patients on clonidine, and clonidine should not be stopped abruptly as it is associated with rebound hypertension. Some pragmatic measures may need to be taken to accommodate care in the case of a patient being involuntarily discharged because his or her presence in the clinic was considered dangerous. For example, office visits may need to be limited to certain times of day, or arrangements may need to be made for dispensing at a community-based pharmacy and conducting UDS collections in a community laboratory. Prescriptions may be faxed to the community-based pharmacy. However, it is not recommended that such arrangements continue indefinitely. A patient in this situation should be encouraged to engage with another health care professional or mutual aid group for counselling and support if possible.

TRANSFER OF CARE TO ANOTHER PHYSICIAN OR CLINIC

There are various reasons why the care of a patient may need to be transferred to another provider, including a breakdown of the doctor-patient relationship, unhealthy relationships with other staff in the clinic, or patient preference due to job or home relocation.

The process for transferring an MMT patient follows the same general guidelines as any transfer of patient care, with the additional requirement of ensuring that no methadone doses are missed due to the transfer:

- Complete and sign the appropriate form for the CPSO to initiate the transfer.
- Make sure your prescription ends about five to seven days after the patient's first appointment with the new provider so that the new physician can make all the necessary arrangements to prescribe methadone to this patient.
- Obtain appropriate patient consent to transfer personal health information to the new physician or clinic.
- Conduct a discharge and termination interview if appropriate.

MMT patients who are being transferred to another MMT program should be maintained at their usual dose unless there is a specific reason to reduce the dose.

Methadone tapering

Tapering a patient's methadone dose is part science, part art.

PATIENT INDICATORS FOR SUCCESSFUL TAPERING

Before attempting to taper a patient's methadone treatment, carefully consider the following factors:

- **Abstinence from all drug use.** Patients must be abstinent from all drugs, especially opioids, cocaine, benzodiazepines and alcohol, before methadone is discontinued, to prevent compensatory increase in other drug use.
- **Social stability.** Patients who have integrated into society by engaging in meaningful work (i.e., job, homemaking, and/or school) and who do not live with or socialize with other active drug users are more likely to be successful at withdrawing from methadone. It is also important for patients to have stable housing and good social supports before beginning a taper.
- **Stable mental and physical health.** Patients with stable psychiatric disease (e.g., no recent hospitalizations) and who are in good physical health will tolerate withdrawal from methadone. It is best to avoid tapering off methadone for a patient who is undergoing treatment for hepatitis C, because the flu-like symptoms caused by interferon are easily mistaken for withdrawal and the associated depression can make the tapering process more difficult.

Therefore, tapering for patients with hepatitis C should be deferred until treatment is complete. Patients undergoing liver transplants should not be tapered while on the waiting list because of the risk of relapse, which would result in the loss of their place on the waiting list. Since stress is a determinant of relapse, especially in late recovery, patients with high levels of ongoing stress (e.g., as the result of the loss of a loved one or serious financial problems) should also delay the tapering process until they have developed a healthy way to cope with these situations.

- **High self-esteem.** Patients with high self-esteem and confidence in their ability to resist cravings are more likely to succeed and tolerate any withdrawal they experience.
- **Pregnancy status.** Tapering is not recommended for women during pregnancy, especially during the first trimester (up to 12 weeks) and the third trimester (at or over 28 weeks), because of the risk of inducing a miscarriage or premature labour, respectively. (See Chapter 15 for more on pregnancy and opioid use.)

Physicians should periodically explore the question of tapering off methadone with any patients who meet the above criteria, but should never force patients to taper if they are not motivated to stop MMT.

SYMPTOMS ASSOCIATED WITH TAPERING

Withdrawal symptoms during tapering

The Short Opiate Withdrawal Scale, or SOWS (Gossop, 1990), reproduced in Table 10-1, is a tool to help physicians rate the severity of withdrawal that patients experience during the tapering process. It should ideally be administered daily, just before the patient is medicated for the day (when methadone levels are at their lowest), to make sure the taper is tolerable. Most patients should score 0 on this scale—that is, they should not report any cravings or thoughts of using of drugs.

TABLE 10-1

Short Opiate Withdrawal Scale (SOWS)

SYMPTOMS	SCORE
Feeling sick	________
Stomach cramps	________
Muscle spasms or twitching	________
Feelings of coldness	________
Heart pounding	________
Muscular tension	________
Aches and pains	________
Yawning	________
Runny/watery eyes	________
Insomnia/problems sleeping	________

Key to scoring 0 not present 1 mild 2 moderate 3 severe

(Reprinted from *Addictive Behaviors, 15* (5), Michael Gossop, The development of a short opiate withdrawal scale, 487–490, copyright 1990, with permission from Elsevier.)

Mood and affective states

Methadone tapering may be associated with a protracted organic mood syndrome. A study of 24 MMT patients who were voluntarily tapering off their methadone reported that some experienced insomnia, depression and anxiety. Sometimes these symptoms lasted for months after completion of the taper. The intensity of the dysphoria was a predictor of the likelihood of relapse (Kanof et al., 1993).

Detoxification fear

Some MMT patients experience "detoxification fear," an anxiety about anticipated withdrawal symptoms during the methadone taper process (Milby, 1988; Milby et al., 1986). A randomized trial showed that MMT patients who are provided with information about tapering and support during their taper experience fewer with-drawal symptoms and are more likely to be successful in terminating MMT (Green & Gossop, 1988).

Use of placebo

Some patients who are voluntarily undergoing the tapering process prefer not to know exactly when they will be given their last dose of methadone. With their consent, these patients may be given placebo (for example, fruit juice with some quinine) for a period of several weeks.

Such use of a placebo should always be discussed beforehand with the patient.

POST-TERMINATION INSTRUCTIONS AND FOLLOW-UP

After the methadone taper is complete, it is advisable to monitor the patient's progress for a time. It is also very important that the patient be educated about the loss of tolerance and the risk of overdose in the case of a relapse. The physician should provide health education about sharing drug paraphernalia and the risk of infectious diseases, and should discuss the importance of immediate follow-up if the patient experiences a relapse or notices the development of another dependency, such as an increase in the consumption of alcohol.

Many patients fear disclosing the occurrence of a relapse to their doctor. Therefore, it is crucial for physicians to create an atmosphere of understanding, to explore this fear with patients ahead of time, and to make clear their willingness to reinstate treatment if necessary. Patients should also be advised to enrol in mutual aid groups to help them on their journey of recovery. Some patients benefit from periodic urine drug screening to help them stay sober. In extremely rare circumstances, patients will agree to start naltrexone to maintain a drug-free state.

References

Cushman, P. Jr. (1978). Methadone maintenance: Long-term follow-up of detoxified patients. *Annals of the New York Academy of Sciences, 311*, 165–172.

Cushman, P. Jr. (1981). Detoxification after methadone maintenance treatment. *Annals of the New York Academy of Sciences, 362*, 217–230.

Dole, V.P. & Nyswander, M.E. (1976). Methadone maintenance treatment: A ten-year perspective. *Journal of the American Medical Association, 235* (19), 2117–2119.

Eklund, C., Hiltunen, A.J., Lennart, M. & Borg, S. (1995). Factors associated with successful withdrawal from methadone maintenance treatment in Sweden. *International Journal of the Addictions, 30*, 1335–1353.

Gossop, M. (1990). The Development of a short opiate withdrawal scale (SOWS). *Addictive Behaviors, 15* (5), 487–490.

Green, L. & Gossop, M. (1988). Effects of information on the opiate withdrawal syndrome. *British Journal of Addiction, 83* (3), 305–309.

Hayes-Bautista, D.E. (1976). Termination of the patient-practitioner relationship: Divorce, patient style. *Journal of Health and Social Behavior, 17*, 12–21.

Hubbard, R.L., Craddock, S.G. & Anderson, J. (2003). Overview of 5-year follow-up outcomes in the drug abuse treatment outcome studies (DATOS). *Journal of Substance Abuse Treatment, 25*, 125–134.

Kanof, P.D., Aronson, M.J. & Ness, R. (1993). Organic mood syndrome associated with detoxification from methadone maintenance. *American Journal of Psychiatry, 150* (3), 423–428.

Milby, J.B. (1988). Methadone maintenance to abstinence: How many make it? *Journal of Nervous and Mental Disease, 176* (7), 409–422.

Milby, J.B., Gurwitch, R.H., Wiebe, D.J., Ling, W., McLellan, A.T. & Woody, G.E. (1986). Prevalence and diagnostic reliability of methadone maintenance detoxification fear. *American Journal of Psychiatry, 143* (6), 739–743.

Senay, E.C., Dorus, W., Goldberg, F. & Thornton, W. (1977). Withdrawal from methadone maintenance: Rate of withdrawal and expectation. *Archives of General Psychiatry, 34* (3), 361–367.

Stimmel, B., Goldberg, J., Cohen, M. & Rotkopf, E. (1978). Detoxification from methadone maintenance: Risk factors associated with relapse to narcotic use. *Annals of the New York Academy of Sciences, 311* (1), 173–180.

Stokes, T., Dixon-Woods, M. & McKinley, R.K. (2004). Ending the doctor-patient relationship in general practice: A proposed model. *Family Practice, 21*, 507–514.

SECTION IV

Clinical issues in methadone maintenance treatment

CHAPTER 11

Concurrent drug use in methadone patients

This chapter describes how methadone interacts with various other drugs, as well as how to recognize and screen for problem drug use in MMT patients.

Overview

The most common drug used in conjunction with methadone is tobacco. In terms of other drugs of abuse, it is more common for patients on stable methadone doses to use cocaine, alcohol or benzodiazepines than opioids. It is therefore important that methadone-dispensing physicians be familiar with the identification and management of patient use of non-opioid drugs of abuse. The DSM-IV criteria for substance dependence are outlined in Chapter 1.

Tobacco use

PREVALENCE AND EFFECTS

Methadone and nicotine consumption are positively correlated among populations of patients undergoing MMT (Spiga et al., 1998; Frosch et al., 2000; Frosch et al., 2002). One study reported that smoking increased the demand for methadone but not vice versa (Spiga et al., 2005). This finding may be due to the effects of methadone and other opioids on nicotinic acetylcholine receptors. In a qualitative study of methadone users, many respondents said that they found smoking and drug use to be complementary—that each helped mitigate the side-effects of the other. Patients were able to recognize the similarity between tobacco smoking and drug use, in that both involved drug cues and could lead to withdrawal symptoms. Patients were also aware that cigarette smoking did not have the kind of immediate negative effects that drug use does.

Nevertheless, smoking does contribute to mortality and morbidity among people who are opiate dependent (Hurt et al., 1996), and there is evidence that many want to quit (Richter et al., 2005; Nahvi et al., 2006).

Tobacco use kills between one-third and one-half of its users (Jha et al., 2002). Every year, about 45,000 Canadians die from tobacco-related diseases—cardiac and cancer mortality lead the list of causes, followed by COPD (chronic obstructive pulmonary disease) (Makomaski Illing & Kaiserman, 2004). Although the prevalence of tobacco use in the general Canadian population has declined to less than 20 per cent (CTUMS, 2005), it is almost two to three times higher among opioid-dependent patients (Frosch et al., 2000; Richter et al., 2001; Richter et al., 2004).

Most patients in MMT programs are unable to stop smoking spontaneously, and require assistance (Richter et al., 2001). Although MMT staff report that they view smoking cessation as important, most do not promote it with their patients (Richter et al., 2005). Staff often feel that patients are unwilling or unable to quit smoking (Richter et al., 2004; McCool et al., 2005). However, a recent study found that 48 per cent of patients who smoked while in an MMT program were contemplating quitting smoking (Nahvi et al., 2006), a finding that matches that of an earlier study (Frosch et al., 1998). Therefore, physicians should follow the guidelines for tobacco treatment with all patients entering MMT (Fiore, 2000).

The standard "5A" approach to treating tobacco dependence calls for health professionals to do the following in all cases:

- ask patients about their smoking status,
- advise patients who smoke to quit,

- assess their readiness to quit,
- assist them according to their readiness, and
- arrange for their progress to be monitored.

Patients most likely to quit are those who are older, have low levels of nicotine dependence, and are not using other drugs. MMT patients who smoke fewer than 10 cigarettes per day or who can go for many hours without smoking are likely to respond to behavioural treatments, whereas pharmacotherapy should be used in patients who smoke 10 or more cigarettes per day.

TREATING PATIENTS WHO ARE READY TO QUIT

Patients who are ready to quit smoking should:

- set a quit date,
- get social support,
- make their homes smoke-free,
- use pharmacotherapy (either NRT and/or bupropion) if indicated, and
- discuss the decision with the attending physician.

Patients who smoke need to prepare practical strategies to avoid their triggers and develop coping skills to prevent lapses and relapses. The effectiveness of nicotine replacement therapy (NRT) increases when contingency management is added to the protocol (Frosch et al., 2002). Moreover, research has shown that when patients were able to quit smoking, they were also able to quit opioid and cocaine use. In a small open-label study, both NRT and bupropion together helped patients quit smoking (Richter et al., 2005). Many patients who smoke crack find that cigarettes and cigarette ash act as triggers for them. Quitting smoking can help reduce their cravings for crack as well.

The nicotine patch can be started at 21 mg per day for six weeks followed by 14 mg for two weeks and 7 mg for two weeks. At the end of the first two weeks, if the patient is smoking while using NRT, it may be necessary to provide combination therapy with immediate-release products such as gum or an inhaler for breakthrough cravings (Karnath, 2002). Bupropion should be used with caution, especially with patients who use cocaine, because both are sympathomimetics and can cause seizures.

TREATING PATIENTS WHO ARE NOT READY TO QUIT

Many patients who smoke are resistant to quitting smoking. Motivational strategies are recommended to help such patients move through the stages of change. Barriers to quitting may include comorbid mood disorder, household or workplace smoking, or lack of funds for stop-smoking medication. It is important for physicians to help patients address any such barriers they face and periodically assess their readiness to move forward.

It may be appropriate to discuss harm reduction, especially with patients who are unable to quit and are beginning to experience a smoking-related disease (Etter et al., 2002; Abdullah, 2005). Since most of the health effects of smoking are not attributable to nicotine, chronic nicotine replacement may be an option for such patients (Zellweger, 2001; Sims & Fiore, 2002).

To conclude, tobacco dependence is an addiction that should be treated like any other: a chronic, relapsing, remitting disease that responds to interventions and treatments by health care providers.

Alcohol use

PREVALENCE AND EFFECTS

Problem drinking and alcohol dependence are common among methadone patients. For example, one retrospective study of 1,700 MMT patients found that 28 per cent consumed more than three drinks per day (Backmund et al., 2003).

Alcohol exacerbates depression and anxiety, may serve as a trigger for cocaine use and accelerates hepatitis C–induced liver damage (Novick, 2000). It contributes to substance-induced mood, anxiety and sleep disorders. Acute alcohol intoxication contributes to methadone-induced sedation; chronic alcohol consumption lowers methadone levels through enzyme induction.

SCREENING AND IDENTIFICATION

All methadone patients should be asked about their alcohol consumption at baseline and at least yearly. Questions should include information about both typical weekly consumption and maximum daily consumption, (e.g., "What's the most you've had to drink on any one day in the past three months?"). Responses should be recorded in terms of a standard drink (i.e., 12 oz. of 5 per cent beer, 5 oz. of table wine, or 1 1/2 oz. of liquor).

Screening questionnaires

Several questionnaires exist to help with evaluating patients' alcohol use.

The CAGE questionnaire, presented in Table 11-1, consists of four short questions (the initial letters of a key word in each question form the title). It has a sensitivity of between 45 and 90 per cent (Fiellin et al., 2000), and can be incorporated into a comprehensive annual assessment. One Yes response is considered a positive screen for women, two for men (Bradley et al., 1998). It is retrospective, so a positive CAGE could indicate a past drinking problem rather than a current drinking problem.

TABLE 11-1

CAGE questions

Have you ever felt you ought to **CUT DOWN** on your drinking?

Have people **ANNOYED** you by criticizing your drinking?

Have you ever felt bad or **GUILTY** about your drinking?

Have you ever had a drink first thing in the morning to steady your nerves or get rid of a hangover (an **"EYE OPENER"**)?

Reproduced with permission from J.A. Ewing, Detecting alcoholism: The CAGE questionnaire, *Journal of the American Medical Association*, 1984; 252:1905–1907.

The 10-item AUDIT questionnaire (Alcohol Use Disorders Identification Test), presented in Table 11-2 (Bush et al., 1998), asks about amount consumed and measures the severity of drinking. A score of 8 or more suggests that the patient may have a drinking problem, while a score of 20 or more suggests that the patient is likely alcohol dependent.

TABLE 11-2

AUDIT questionnaire

Instructions: The 10 items below refer to how you have behaved during the past year. For each item, indicate the statement that is most true for you by circling the appropriate number next to the item. Then total your scores for all 10 questions.

Note: If you suspect that you have a drinking or drug problem you should seek help from a health professional regardless of how you score on this screening test.

DRINK DEFINITIONS

Some items below ask questions about how many drinks you have had. For the purpose of this screening test, a drink is defined as follows:

- a single small glass of beer (8 oz., or 1/2 pint), or
- a single shot/measure of liquor/spirits, or
- a single glass of wine (5 oz.).

1. How often do you have a drink containing alcohol?

⓪ Never
① Monthly or less
② 2 to 4 times per month
③ 2 to 3 times per week
④ 4 or more times per week

Continued on next page

TABLE 11-2: AUDIT QUESTIONNAIRE (continued)

2. How many drinks containing alcohol do you have on a typical day when you are drinking? (Make sure you understand how each drink is defined—see "Drink definitions," above.)

⓪ 1 or 2
① 3 or 4
② 5 or 6
③ 7, 8 or 9
④ 10 or more

3. How often do you have 6 or more drinks on one occasion?

⓪ Never
① Less than monthly
② Monthly
③ Weekly
④ Daily or almost daily

4. How often during the last year have you found that you were not able to stop drinking once you had started?

⓪ Never
① Less than monthly
② Monthly
③ Weekly
④ Daily or almost daily

5. How often during the last year have you failed to do what was normally expected from you because of drinking?

⓪ Never
① Less than monthly
② Monthly
③ Weekly
④ Daily or almost daily

6. How often during the last year have you needed a first drink in the morning to get yourself going after a heavy drinking session?

⓪ Never
① Less than monthly
② Monthly
③ Weekly
④ Daily or almost daily

7. How often during the last year have you had a feeling of guilt or remorse after drinking?

⓪ Never
① Less than monthly
② Monthly
③ Weekly
④ Daily or almost daily

8. How often during the last year have you been unable to remember what happened the night before because you had been drinking?

⓪ Never
① Less than monthly
② Monthly
③ Weekly
④ Daily or almost daily

9. Have you or someone else been injured as a result of your drinking?

⓪ No
② Yes, but not in the last year
④ Yes, during the last year

10. Has a relative or friend or doctor or other health worker been concerned about your drinking or suggested you cut down?

⓪ No
② Yes, but not in the last year
④ Yes, during the last year

Laboratory markers

Laboratory tests for GGT (gamma glutamyl transferase) and MCV (mean cell volume) can be used to confirm a diagnosis of alcohol dependence and monitor response to treatment. These tests have a sensitivity of 35 to 60 per cent for detecting heavy alcohol consumption (Girella et al., 1994; Wetterling et al., 1998). Methadone-prescribing physicians must be able to distinguish hepatic abnormalities caused by hepatitis C from those caused by alcohol, as illustrated in Table 11-3 on page 96.

Common presentations of heavy drinking in MMT patients

Depression, anxiety, insomnia and family dysfunction are extremely common among methadone patients. MMT physicians sometimes focus on opioid and cocaine use without considering alcohol as a potential cause of these problems.

Other common presentations of heavy alcohol consumption include worsening liver function, trauma and gastritis.

The at-risk or problem drinker

Most heavy drinkers do not meet the criteria for alcohol dependence but are considered to be "at-risk drinkers" (see Table 11-4 on page 96): they do not experience alcohol withdrawal, they abstain or drink moderately as the occasion warrants, and their consumption has not caused severe social or physical consequences (Kahan et al., 1995).

Brief advice protocol for at-risk drinkers

Controlled trials have demonstrated that brief advice from a physician is effective in reducing alcohol consumption, injuries, emergency-room visits, hospital days and health care costs in problem drinkers (Fleming et al., 1997; Manwell et al., 2000; Fleming et al., 2000; Ockene et al., 1999; Senft et al., 1997).

The following protocol is recommended:

- Inform the patient of the low-risk guidelines (14 drinks per week for men, nine for women; no more than two drinks per drinking day), emphasizing that patients on MMT should aim for considerably less than this because alcohol enhances the sedating effects of methadone. Patients with hepatitis C should not exceed two drinks per week.
- Link the patient's health condition to his or her alcohol consumption. Point out that almost all alcohol-related conditions improve substantially within weeks of beginning abstinence or reducing drinking. For MMT patients, the most common alcohol-related concerns will likely be depression, anxiety, insomnia, financial problems, family dysfunction and liver damage from hepatitis C.
- Monitor GGT and MCV at baseline and monthly, and inform the patient of the results. Monitor AST and ALT if the patient has hepatitis C.
- Ask the patient to set a treatment goal; for example, abstinence or reduced drinking. If the goal is reduced drinking, ask the patient to specify a goal in terms of a number of drinks per day and a number of days per week.
- Ask the patient to keep a daily record of the number of drinks consumed and to bring it in at each office visit.
- Suggest strategies for reducing alcohol consumption and avoiding intoxication (see Table 11-5 on page 97).
- Arrange follow-up visits.
- If the patient doesn't respond to brief advice, consider referral for more intensive treatment.

TABLE 11-3

Distinguishing between hepatitis C and heavy alcohol consumption as causes of hepatic abnormalities

	HEPATITIS C	ALCOHOL
GGT	Usually normal[1]	Often elevated[2]
AST	ALT > AST	AST:ALT = 2:1
MCV	Usually normal[3]	Often elevated[4]

TABLE 11-4

At-risk drinking versus alcohol dependence

	AT-RISK DRINKING	ALCOHOL DEPENDENCE
Withdrawal symptoms[5]	none	often
Tolerance	mild	marked
Weekly consumption	above low-risk guidelines	40–60 drinks per week or more
Drinks fewer than four drinks day	often	rarely
Social consequences[6]	none or mild	often severe
Physical consequences[7]	none or mild	often severe
Socially stable	usually	often not
Neglect of major responsibilities	no	yes

1 Except in hepatitis C–induced cirrhosis.
2 GGT is also elevated by diabetes, obesity, enzyme-inducing medications such as phenytoin, and obstructive liver disease.
3 Except in hepatitis C–induced cirrhosis.
4 MCV is also elevated by hypothyroidism, liver disease, B12 or folate deficiency and medications such as valproic acid.
5 In almost all cases, the presence of withdrawal symptoms indicates alcohol dependence.
6 Examples of mild: occasional argument with spouse, fatigue at work. Examples of severe: loss of family or job.
7 Examples of mild: hypertension, insomnia, fatty liver. Examples of severe: cirrhosis, pancreatitis

TABLE 11-5

Strategies for avoiding intoxication

Drink no more than one standard drink per hour.
Sip drinks, don't gulp.
Drink on a full stomach.
Dilute drinks with mixer.
Alternate alcoholic with non-alcoholic drinks.
Take a 20-minute "time-out" between deciding to have a drink and taking the drink.

TREATING ALCOHOL DEPENDENCE

Counselling

The most important aspect of treatment is counselling. MMT patients will reduce their alcohol consumption in response to counselling (Bradley et al., 1998), yet on average, alcohol use does not decline when patients are started on methadone (Novick, 2000; Fiellin et al., 2000; Srivastava et al., 2007). This suggests that MMT patients who are at-risk drinkers or alcohol dependent are inadequately identified and counselled.

Anti-craving medications

Several medications exist that have been shown in controlled trials to reduce the frequency and intensity of alcohol consumption in alcohol-dependent patients. These medications are generally safe and non-addicting, and are probably under-prescribed. Research is under way to determine which combinations of anti-craving medications are effective and which patient sub-populations respond best.

Topiramate has been shown in several controlled trials to reduce alcohol consumption. The trials used a mean dose of 300 mg per day, which is the standard anticonvulsant dose (Johnson et al., 2003). Acamprosate antagonizes glutamate, relieving protracted withdrawal symptoms and craving (Mason, 2001). Naltrexone is contraindicated in methadone patients because it is an opioid antagonist and will trigger severe withdrawal.

Disulfiram is useful in highly motivated, stable patients who take it under the supervision of a spouse or family member. It inhibits acetaldehyde dehydrogenase, so patients must not drink alcohol while taking disulfiram or they will experience toxicity from the accumulation of acetaldehyde. Symptoms include vomiting, flushed face and headache. Disulfiram can cause death through hypotension and arrhythmias in patients who have underlying cardiovascular disease or are on antihypertensive medications. Disulfiram is contraindicated in pregnancy and should be avoided by patients with severe heart disease, psychosis, severe depression or severe liver disease.

An added benefit of disulfiram is that several controlled trials have found it reduces cocaine use in MMT patients (Petrakis, 2000).

Alcohol use and take-home methadone doses

Patients who present to the pharmacy intoxicated should have their dose held until they are alert. Physicians should exercise caution in granting take-home dose privileges to heavy drinkers because the combination of alcohol excess and methadone can be dangerous.

ALCOHOL WITHDRAWAL

Alcohol withdrawal begins six to 12 hours after an alcohol-dependent person's last drink and resolves within three to seven days. Physical signs include postural and intention tremor, ataxia, diaphoresis, tachycardia and hypertension. Complications include seizures, arrhythmias, hallucinations and delirium.

Withdrawal should be suspected if the patient reports daily consumption of six or more drinks per day, if drinking begins at a predictable time in the morning or afternoon, if the patient reports morning anxiety or tremor, or if the patient has a past history of seizures.

Benzodiazepines are the first-line treatment for alcohol withdrawal (Mayo-Smith 1997; Holbrook Crowther et al., 1999).

The severity of withdrawal should be measured using the CIWA-A (Clinical Institute Withdrawal Assessment for Alcohol), a validated and widely used instrument shown in Table 11-6. A score of 10 or more indicates the need for benzodiazepine treatment. Treatment is considered to be completed when the patient scores less than 8 on two consecutive readings and feels comfortable, with minimal postural tremor.

TABLE 11-6

Clinical Institute Withdrawal Assessment for Alcohol (CIWA-A)

NAUSEA AND VOMITING

Ask, "Do you feel sick to your stomach? Have you vomited?"

Observation:

0 no nausea and no vomiting

1

2

3

4 intermittent nausea with dry heaves

5

6

7 constant nausea, frequent dry heaves and vomiting

AGITATION

Observation:

0 normal activity

1 somewhat more than normal activity

2

3

4 moderately fidgety and restless

5

6

7 paces back and forth during most of the interview, or constantly thrashes about

Continued on next page

TABLE 11-6: CLINICAL INSTITUTE WITHDRAWAL ASSESSMENT FOR ALCOHOL (CIWA-A) (continued)

TREMOR

Arms extended and fingers spread apart.

Observation:

0 no tremor

1 not visible, but can be felt fingertip to fingertip

2

3

4 moderate with patient's arms extended

5

6

7 severe, even with arms not extended

TACTILE DISTURBANCES

Ask, "Have you any itching, 'pins and needles' sensations, burning or numbness, or do you feel as if bugs are crawling on your skin?"

Observation:

0 none

1 very mild itching, pins and needles, burning or numbness

2 mild itching, pins and needles, burning or numbness

3 moderate itching, pins and needles, burning or numbness

4 moderately severe hallucinations

5 severe hallucinations

6 extremely severe hallucinations

7 continuous hallucinations

PAROXYSMAL SWEATS

Observation:

0 no sweat visible

1 barely perceptible sweating, palms moist

2

3

4 beads of sweat obvious on forehead

5

6

7 drenching sweats

AUDITORY DISTURBANCES

Ask, "Are you more aware of sounds around you? Are they harsh? Do they frighten you? Are you hearing anything that is disturbing to you? Are you hearing things you know are not there?"

Observation:

0 not present

1 very mild harshness or ability to frighten

2 mild harshness or ability to frighten

3 moderate harshness or ability to frighten

4 moderately severe hallucinations

5 severe hallucinations

6 extremely severe hallucinations

7 continuous hallucinations

Continued on next page

TABLE 11-6: CLINICAL INSTITUTE WITHDRAWAL ASSESSMENT FOR ALCOHOL (CIWA-A) (continued)

ANXIETY

Ask, "Do you feel nervous?"

Observation:

0 no anxiety, at ease

1 mildly anxious

2

3

4 moderately anxious (or guarded, so anxiety is inferred)

5

6

7 equivalent to acute panic states as seen in severe delirium or acute schizophrenic reactions

VISUAL DISTURBANCES

Ask, "Does the light appear to be too bright? Is its colour different? Does it hurt your eyes? Are you seeing anything that is disturbing to you? Are you seeing things you know are not there?"

Observation:

0 not present

1 very mild sensitivity

2 mild sensitivity

3 moderate sensitivity

4 moderately severe sensitivity

5 severe hallucinations

6 extremely severe hallucinations

7 continuous hallucinations

HEADACHE, FULLNESS IN HEAD

Ask, "Does your head feel different? Does it feel like there is a band around your head?" Do not rate for dizziness or light-headedness. Otherwise, rate severity.

Observation:

0 not present

1 very mild

2 mild

3 moderate

4 moderately severe

5 severe

6 very severe

7 extremely severe

ORIENTATION AND CLOUDING OF SENSORIUM

Ask, "What day is this? Where are you? Who am I?"

Observation:

0 oriented—knows date (and can do serial additions)

1 is uncertain about date (or cannot do serial additions)

2 disoriented for date by no more than two calendar days

3 disoriented for date by more than two calendar days

4 disoriented for place and/or person

(Sullivan et al., 1989; Reoux & Miller, 2000)

TREATMENT OF WITHDRAWAL

Patients not yet on methadone

Patients who are dependent on both alcohol and opioids should be withdrawn safely from alcohol and abstinent for at least several days before they begin MMT. It can be dangerous to use large doses of benzodiazepines for alcohol withdrawal management while initiating MMT (see Chapter 4 for more on the pharmacology of methadone). Patients with dual dependencies should also be warned that relapsing to alcohol use during methadone initiation can cause methadone toxicity. In patients with severe alcohol withdrawal and opioid dependence, titration at an inpatient treatment facility should be considered.

Patients on methadone

Because of the risk of methadone-benzodiazepine toxicity, alcohol withdrawal is best treated in an inpatient or emergency-department setting. Lorazepam may be safer than diazepam in methadone patients because it has a shorter duration of action and is not metabolized to active metabolites in the liver (Peppers, 1996). Lorazepam (see detailed protocol in Table 11-7) is particularly advised for patients on higher methadone doses, for elderly patients and for those with cirrhosis, as well as for use during the methadone induction phase. If the patient's withdrawal is mild and improving, it is best to withhold benzodiazepines and observe, in order to avoid mixed methadone-benzodiazepine toxicity.

Whenever possible, patients should be observed for 12 to 24 hours after their last benzodiazepine dose. A patient who is drowsy should be admitted and monitored closely. A patient who remains alert should be sent home with a responsible friend or family member, or to the local withdrawal management service. The patient should be reassessed the next day, before receiving a methadone dose.

Cocaine use

PREVALENCE AND EFFECTS

Cocaine abuse and dependence are very common among methadone patients. Cocaine use often declines when patients start methadone, although not to the same degree as opioid use (Faggiano et al., 2003; Gossop et al., 2003).

TABLE 11-7

Lorazepam protocol for alcohol withdrawal

Lorazepam SL, po1–2 mg q2 –4 H until symptoms abate, or CIWA≤10.

Treatment is completed when patient is comfortable with minimal tremor, or CIWA < 8 on two consecutive readings.

Observe for 12 to 24 hours before discharge.

Thiamine 100 mg IM, then 100 mg po for three days.

If history of seizures: lorazepam 2 mg for at least four doses.

Admit if patient:

- still shows marked withdrawal despite 8–10 mg lorazepam
- shows evidence of complications (seizures, arrhythmias, DTs
- is dehydrated, has electrolyte abnormalities or is medically ill.

Pharmacology

Cocaine blocks presynaptic uptake of dopamine, epinephrine and norepinephrine. It is either injected or smoked as crack (cocaine mixed with sodium bicarbonate). It causes a brief but intense euphoria, often followed by paranoia and agitation.

SCREENING AND IDENTIFICATION

Cocaine and its metabolite can be reliably detected with urine drug screening (see Chapter 8 for a detailed discussion of urine drug screening). Physical signs include weight loss and track marks.

Medical complications

Acute cocaine intoxication can cause seizures, delirium and psychosis. It also causes vasospasm, arrhythmias and hypertension, which can result in myocardial infarction, stroke and other cardiovascular events. Injection cocaine use is a vector for hepatitis C and HIV infection.

Psychological complications

The consequences of cocaine use include depression, anxiety, suicide, violence and drug-induced paranoia and psychosis.

Withdrawal

Withdrawal is primarily psychological. In the first one or two days after a cocaine binge, the user sleeps deeply (the "crash" phase). This is followed by several weeks of depression, irritability, strong cravings and insomnia.

TREATING COCAINE DEPENDENCE

No medication has yet been shown to be effective in treating cocaine dependence, although research continues (Petrakis et al., 2000). Patients who use cocaine should be encouraged to participate in treatment options such as counselling.

Cocaine use and take-home methadone doses

Patients on MMT should not be granted take-home dose privileges if they are actively using cocaine, because they are at greater risk for methadone abuse, overdose and diversion. Contingency management (giving take-home doses for urine samples free of cocaine) has been shown to be effective in reducing cocaine use.

Cannabis use

PREVALENCE AND EFFECTS

Cannabis use is extremely common among people taking methadone. Its use is not associated with poor outcomes for MMT except in those patients that meet criteria for cannabis dependence (Epstein & Preston, 2003).

SCREENING AND IDENTIFICATION

Regular cannabis use can be detected for up to 30 days on an immunoassay, but routine long-term weekly urine screening for cannabis is probably not justified. If the patient's goal is to stop use then periodic screening can be used to detect relapse. However, given the long duration of detection, the results should be interpreted in light of the clinical situation to make sure the test is not detecting remote use. The harm from smoked marijuana is beginning to be described, especially in chronic daily smokers, and therefore physicians should not condone its use as a "lesser of two evils."

Pharmacology

Cannabis causes relaxation and a feeling of well-being, accompanied by mild hallucinogenic effects such as perceptual distortions. Withdrawal is not clinically significant.

There is currently little evidence to support the therapeutic use of smoked cannabis (Gurley et al., 1998; Watson et al., 2000).

Psychological complications

Cannabis should be avoided in patients with a significant Axis I mental illness (as defined in the DSM-IV). It can induce depression, psychosis and schizophrenia in predisposed patients (Hambrecht & Hafner, 2000). Cannabis dependence can contribute to depression and family dysfunction.

CANNABIS DEPENDENCE

Cannabis dependence should be suspected in patients who are heavy daily cannabis users, particularly if they present with depression, anxiety, psychosis or social dysfunction. As with cocaine, there are currently no medications that have been approved for the treatment of cannabis dependence. Urine drug screening can be used for treatment monitoring and contingency management, and patients should receive counselling.

Benzodiazepine use

PREVALENCE AND EFFECTS

Benzodiazepine misuse and dependence are common in methadone patients and are associated with greater drug use and psychopathology (Bleich et al., 1999; Bleich et al., 2002). Benzodiazepines impair cognition and induce euphoria in MMT patients (Farre et al., 1998; Spiga et al., 2001). Patients who have been prescribed both methadone and diazepam are more likely to experience both accidental and deliberate overdoses than patients prescribed either drug alone (Man et al., 2004).

Benzodiazepines increase the risk of depression, falls and motor vehicle accidents, and benzodiazepine withdrawal can cause seizures, psychosis and delirium. Because of these risks and the availability of effective alternatives, benzodiazepines are no longer considered the first-line medication for mood or anxiety disorders (Asnis et al., 2004; Allgulander et al., 2003; Van Ameringen et al., 2003).

Tolerance and dependence

Tolerance to the hypnotic (sleep-inducing) effects of benzodiazepines develops within weeks, whereas tolerance to their anxiolytic effects develops very slowly, if at all. Diazepam, lorazepam and alprazolam have the highest abuse liability, while oxazepam, clonazepam and chlordiazepoxide have the lowest.

Benzodiazepine dependence shares the same clinical features as dependence on other substances, including loss of control over substance use and continued use despite adverse consequences. As with opioids, withdrawal resulting from cessation of benzodiazepines does not in itself indicate psychological dependence.

Withdrawal

Withdrawal can occur, even with therapeutic doses, after daily benzodiazepine use of from one to two months. It is more severe with high doses or short-acting agents, after a long duration of use or in the presence of an underlying anxiety disorder. The onset of withdrawal takes place from one to four days after the last dose, depending on the duration of action of the benzodiazepine. Withdrawal presents with both anxiety-related symptoms (panic attacks, insomnia and irritability) and neurological symptoms (harsh sounds, tinnitus and blurry or distorted vision) (Marriott & Tyrer, 1993). Abrupt cessation of 50 mg of diazepam or its equivalent can result in seizures, psychosis, delirium, arrhythmias and hypertension. The sub-acute phase of withdrawal can take several weeks or months to resolve.

Screening and identification

A patient's family physician can provide valuable information about whether he or she is showing behaviours suggesting benzodiazepine abuse or dependence (see also Chapter 8 for information about urine drug screening).

MANAGEMENT OF MMT PATIENTS WHO USE BENZODIAZEPINES

Overview of benzodiazepine tapering

Physician support and cognitive therapy have been shown to be effective in benzodiazepine tapering (Bashir et al., 1994; Baillargeon et al., 2003; Morgan et al., 2002; Spiegel, 1999). Periodic attempts to taper are warranted even if the patient is taking therapeutic doses with no apparent adverse effects—tapering the dose may lead to the patient feeling more alert and energetic, and better able to engage in counselling (Rickels et al., 1990; Ashton, 1994).

Physicians should explore these benefits of tapering with patients, and discuss withdrawal symptoms. There is usually no need to quickly discontinue therapeutic benzodiazepine use, and slow tapers work better than fast tapers. Doses should be scheduled rather than issued as needed.

Slow, halt or reverse the taper if the patient experiences severe anxiety or depression. Provide follow-up every one to four weeks, depending on the rate of the taper.

Patients who are tapering their benzodiazepine use should be encouraged to become active, rely on their social networks for support and use stress-reduction techniques. Adjunctive agents such as mood stabilizers and antidepressants may be considered if the taper is difficult (Ansseau & De Roeck, 1993; Harris et al., 2000), although further study is needed on their effectiveness. Patients with an underlying depression may experience increased anxiety and suicidal ideation during the taper; halt or reverse the taper if this occurs.

Opioid- and benzodiazepine-dependent patients not yet on methadone

Patients who present with both opioid and benzodiazepine dependence should be admitted to an inpatient setting and tapered off benzodiazepines prior to initiating methadone treatment. Concurrent methadone initiation and high-dose benzodiazepine tapering can cause an overdose because it is impossible to determine the patient's benzodiazepine use and tolerance until the taper is well under way.

MMT patients on stable, moderate benzodiazepine doses

It is probably safest to taper benzodiazepine doses for MMT patients with lorazepam or clonazepam rather than a long-acting agent such as diazepam. Diazepam may cause excessive and prolonged sedation in methadone patients, particularly if they are older or have severe liver or respiratory disease. For patients on alprazolam or triazolam, the taper should use alprazolam, triazolam or an equivalent dose of clonazepam (Harrison et al., 1984; Albeck, 1987).

The patient should be "converted" to no more than the equivalent dose of the new agent, in divided doses. It might be safest to start the patient on a dose slightly lower than the equivalent, particularly if you are uncertain about his or her level of compliance. Equivalence tables are approximate; adjust the initial dose according to symptoms. Taper by no more than 5 mg diazepam equivalent per week and adjust the rate of the taper as symptoms indicate. Slow the pace of the taper once the dose is below the equivalent of 20 mg of diazepam. Dispense daily, twice weekly or weekly depending on dose and patient reliability. The most convenient strategy is to dispense the benzodiazepine along with the patient's methadone.

MMT patients who are abusing high doses of benzodiazepines

Inpatient medically managed withdrawal should be considered in patients taking high doses, such as 50 mg of diazepam equivalent or more. The clinician should keep in mind that benzodiazepine withdrawal has a more gradual course than alcohol withdrawal, so there is time to adjust the dose if the patient is becoming worse. Also, the risks of combined methadone-benzodiazepine toxicity are much greater than the risks of benzodiazepine withdrawal. Furthermore, it is easy to overestimate a patient's underlying benzodiazepine tolerance, as patients sometimes exaggerate their benzodiazepine use, which can fluctuate widely from day to day.

For these reasons, it is best not to start tapering with a fixed, scheduled dose. The taper should proceed with small to moderate as-needed doses of lorazepam or clonazepam, dispensed every four to six hours. If the patient is doing well on such a dose, it can be maintained and slowly tapered. If the patient becomes anxious or agitated, the dose can be carefully increased until the patient is reasonably comfortable. The optimal daily dose is one that prevents both sedation and marked agitation. That dose should be tapered by no more than 10 per cent per day. The taper may be slowed once a therapeutic dose is reached. If tapering is completed in an outpatient setting, the benzodiazepine should be dispensed daily along with the patient's methadone.

Other drug use

Amphetamines are similar to cocaine in their effects, but are longer acting.

Ecstasy acts on serotonergic neurons to cause feelings of warmth and social disinhibition. The long-term effects of ecstasy use are not fully understood.

GHB (gamma-hydroxybutyrate) is a sedating drug with effects similar to those of barbiturates. Heavy, daily use of GHB can cause a severe withdrawal syndrome similar to barbiturate withdrawal, with seizures, delirium and psychosis. GHB withdrawal is treated with tapering doses of phenobarbital.

Hallucinogens such as LSD and mescaline can trigger psychosis in predisposed individuals.

References

Abdullah, A.S. (2005). How far should we promote smoking reduction in order to promote smoking cessation? *Asian Pacific Journal of Cancer Prevention, 6* (2), 231–234.

Albeck, J.H. (1987). Withdrawal and detoxification from benzodiazepine dependence: A potential role for clonazepam. *Journal of Clinical Psychiatry, 48* (suppl.), 43–49.

Allgulander, C., Bandelow, B., Hollander, E. Montgomery, S.A., Nutt, D.J., Okasha, A. et al. (2003). WCA recommendations for the long-term treatment of generalized anxiety disorder. *CNS Spectrums, 8* (suppl. 1), 53–61.

Ansseau, M. & De Roeck, J. (1993). Trazodone in benzodiazepine dependence. *Journal of Clinical Psychiatry, 54* (5), 189–191.

Ashton H. (1994). The treatment of benzodiazepine dependence. *Addiction, 89* (11), 1535–1541.

Asnis, G.M., Kohn, S.R., Henderson, M. & Brown, N.L. (2004). SSRIs versus non-SSRIs in post-traumatic stress disorder: An update with recommendations. *Drugs, 64* (4), 383–404.

Backmund, M., Schutz, C.G., Meyer, K., Eichenlaub, D. & Soyka, M. (2003). Alcohol consumption in heroin users, methadone-substituted and codeine-substituted patients: Frequency and correlates of use. *European Addiction Research, 9* (1), 45–50.

Baillargeon, L., Landreville, P., Verreault, R., Beauchemin, J.P., Gregoire, J.P. & Morin, C.M. (2003). Discontinuation of benzodiazepines among older insomniac adults treated with cognitive-behavioural therapy combined with gradual tapering: A randomized trial. *Canadian Medical Association Journal, 169* (10), 1015–1020.

Bashir, K., King, M. & Ashworth, M. (1994). Controlled evaluation of brief intervention by general practitioners to reduce chronic use of benzodiazepines. *British Journal of General Practice, 44* (386), 408–412.

Bleich, A., Gelkopf, M., Schmidt, V., Hayward, R., Bodner, G. & Adelson, M. (1999). Correlates of benzodiazepine abuse in methadone maintenance treatment. A 1-year prospective study in an Israeli clinic. *Addiction, 94* (10), 1533–1540.

Bleich, A., Gelkopf, M., Weizman, T. & Adelson, M. (2002). Benzodiazepine abuse in a methadone maintenance treatment clinic in Israel: Characteristics and a pharmacotherapeutic approach. *Israel Journal of Psychiatry and Related Sciences, 39* (2), 104–112.

Bradley, K.A., Boyd-Wickizer, J., Powell, S.H. & Burman M.L. (1998). Alcohol screening questionnaires in women: A critical review. *Journal of the American Medical Association, 280* (2), 166–171.

Bush, K., Kivlahan, D.R., McDonell, M.B., Fihn, S.D. & Bradley, K.A. (1998). The AUDIT alcohol consumption questions (AUDIT-C): An effective brief screening test for problem drinking. Ambulatory Care Quality Improvement Project (ACQUIP). Alcohol Use Disorders Identification Test. *Archives of Internal Medicine, 158* (16), 1789–1795.

CTUMS (2005). *Canadian Tobacco Use Monitoring Survey*. Health Canada. Health Promotion Directorate; Statistics Canada. Special Surveys Group.

Epstein, D.H. & Preston, K.L. (2003). Does cannabis use predict poor outcome for heroin-dependent patients on maintenance treatment? Past findings and more evidence against. *Addiction, 98* (3), 269–279.

Etter, J.F., Laszlo, E., Zellweger, J.P., Perrot, C. & Perneger, T.V. (2002). Nicotine replacement to reduce cigarette consumption in smokers who are unwilling to quit: A randomized trial. *Journal of Clinical Psychopharmacology, 22* (5), 487–95.

Faggiano, F., Vigna-Taglianti, F., Versino, E. & Lemma, P. (2003). Methadone maintenance at different dosages for opioid dependence. *Cochrane Database of Systematic Reviews, 3,* no. CD002208.

Farre, M., Teran, M.T., Roset, P.N., Mas, M., Torrens, M. & Cami, J. (1998.) Abuse liability of flunitrazepam among methadone-maintained patients. *Psychopharmacology, 140* (4), 486–495.

Fiellin, D.A., Reid, M.C. & O'Connor, P.G. (2000). Screening for alcohol problems in primary care: A systematic review. *Archives of Internal Medicine, 160,* (13), 1977–1989.

Fiore, M., Bailey, W.C., Cohen, S.J., Faith Dorfman, S., Goldstein, M.G., Gritz, E.R. et al., (2000). *Treating Tobacco Use and Dependence. Clinical Practice Guideline*. Rockville, MD: US Department of Health and Human Services, Public Health Services.

Fleming, M., Mundt, M., French, M., Manwell, L., Stauffacher, E. & Barry, K. (2000). Benefit-cost analysis of brief physician advice with problem drinkers in primary care settings. *Medical Care, 38* (1), 7–18.

Fleming, M.F., Barry, K.L., Manwell, L.B., Johnson, K. & London, R. (1997). Brief physician advice for problem alcohol drinkers. A randomized controlled trial in community-based primary care practices. *Journal of the American Medical Association, 277* (13), 1039–1045.

Frosch, D.L., Nahom, D. & Shoptaw, S. (2002). Optimizing smoking cessation outcomes among the methadone maintained. *Journal of Substance Abuse Treatment, 23* (4), 425–430.

Frosch, D.L., Shoptaw, S., Jarvik, M.E., Rawson, R.A. & Ling, W. (1998). Interest in smoking cessation among methadone maintained outpatients. *Journal of Addictive Diseases, 17* (2), 9–19.

Frosch, D.L., Shoptaw, S., Nahom, D. & Jarvik, M.E. (2000). Associations between tobacco smoking and illicit drug use among methadone-maintained opiate-dependent individuals. *Experimental and Clinical Psychopharmacology, 8* (1), 97–103.

Girela, E., Villanueva, E., Hernandez-Cueto, C. & Luna, J.D. (1994) Comparison of the CAGE questionnaire versus some biochemical markers in the diagnosis of alcoholism. *Alcohol, 29* (3), 337–343.

Gossop, M., Marsden, J., Stewart, D. & Kidd, T. (2003). The National Treatment Outcome Research Study (NTORS): 4–5 year follow-up results. *Addiction, 98* (3), 291–303.

Gurley, R.J., Aranow, R. & Katz, M. (1998). Medicinal marijuana: A comprehensive review. *Journal of Psychoactive Drugs, 30* (2), 137–147.

Hambrecht, M. & Hafner, H. (2000). Cannabis, vulnerability, and the onset of schizophrenia: An epidemiological perspective. *Australian and New Zealand Journal of Psychiatry, 34* (3), 468–475.

Harris, J.T., Roache, J.D. & Thornton, J.E. (2000). A role for valproate in the treatment of sedative-hypnotic withdrawal and for relapse prevention. *Alcohol, 35* (4), 319–323.

Harrison, M., Busto, U., Naranjo, C.A., Kaplan, H.L. & Sellers, E.M. (1984). Diazepam tapering in detoxification for high-dose benzodiazepine abuse. *Clinical Pharmacology and Therapeutics, 36* (4), 527–533.

Holbrook, A.M., Crowther, R., Lotter, A., Cheng, C. & King, D. (1999) Meta-analysis of benzodiazepine use in the treatment of acute alcohol withdrawal. *Canadian Medical Association Journal, 160* (5), 649–655.

Hurt, R.D., Offord, K.P., Croghan, I.T., Gomez-Dahl, L., Kottke, T.E., Morse, R.M. et al. (1996). Mortality following inpatient addictions treatment. Role of tobacco use in a community-based cohort. *Journal of the American Medical Association, 275* (14), 1097–1103.

Jha, P., Ranson, M.K. Nguyen, S.N. & Yach, D. (2002). Estimates of global and regional smoking prevalence in 1995, by age and sex. *American Journal of Public Health, 92* (6), 1002–1006.

Johnson, B.A., Ait-Daoud, N., Bowden, C.L., DiClemente, C.C., Roache, J.D., Lawson, K. et al. (2003). Oral topiramate for treatment of alcohol dependence: A randomised controlled trial. *The Lancet, 361* (9370), 1677–1685.

Kahan, M., Wilson, L. & Becker, L. (1995). Effectiveness of physician-based interventions with problem drinkers: A review. *Canadian Medical Association Journal, 152* (6), 851–859.

Karnath, B. (2002). Smoking cessation: The most effective strategies. *Journal of Respiratory Diseases, 23* (10), 496–502.

Makomaski Illing, E.M. & M.J. Kaiserman. (2004). Mortality attributable to tobacco use in Canada and its regions, 1998. *Canadian Journal of Public Health, 95* (1), 38–44.

Man, L.H., Best, D., Gossop, M., Stillwell, G. & Strang, J. (2004). Relationship between prescribing and risk of opiate overdose among drug users in and out of maintenance treatment. *European Addiction Research, 10* (1), 35–40.

Manwell, L.B., Fleming, M.F., Mundt, M.P., Stauffacher, E.A. & Barry, K.L. (2000). Treatment of problem alcohol use in women of childbearing age: Results of a brief intervention trial. *Alcoholism, Clinical and Experimental Research, 24* (10), 1517–1524.

Marriott, S. & Tyrer, P. (1993). Benzodiazepine dependence: Avoidance and withdrawal. *Drug Safety, 9* (2), 93–103.

Mason, B.J. (2001). Treatment of alcohol-dependent outpatients with acamprosate: A clinical review. *Journal of Clinical Psychiatry, 62* (suppl. 20), 42–48.

Mayo-Smith, M.F. (1997). Pharmacological management of alcohol withdrawal: A meta-analysis and evidence-based practice guideline. American Society of Addiction Medicine Working Group on Pharmacological Management of Alcohol Withdrawal. *Journal of the American Medical Association, 278* (2), 144–151.

McCool, R.M., Richter, K.P. & Choi, W.S. (2005). Benefits of and barriers to providing smoking treatment in methadone clinics: Findings from a national study. *American Journal on Addictions, 14* (4), 358–366.

Morgan, J.D., Wright, D.J. & Chrystyn, H. (2002). Pharmacoeconomic evaluation of a patient education letter aimed at reducing long-term prescribing of benzodiazepines. *Pharmacy World and Science, 24* (6), 231–235.

Nahvi, S., Richter, K., Li, X., Modali, L. & Arnsten, J. (2006). Cigarette smoking and interest in quitting in methadone maintenance patients. *Addictive Behaviors, 31* (11), 2006, 2127–2134.

Novick, D.M. (2000). The impact of hepatitis C virus infection on methadone maintenance treatment. *Mount Sinai Journal of Medicine, 67* (5–6), 437–443.

Ockene, J.K., Adams A., Hurley, T.G., Wheeler, E.V. & Hebert, J.R. (1999). Brief physician– and nurse practitioner–delivered counseling for high-risk drinkers: Does it work? *Archives of Internal Medicine, 159* (18), 2198–2205.

Peppers, M.P. (1996). Benzodiazepines for alcohol withdrawal in the elderly and in patients with liver disease. *Pharmacotherapy, 16* (1), 49–57.

Petrakis, I.L., Carroll, K.M., Nich, C., Gordon, L.T., McCance-Katz, E.F., Frankforter, T. et al. (2000). Disulfiram treatment for cocaine dependence in methadone-maintained opioid addicts. *Addiction, 95* (2), 219–228.

Reoux, J.P. & Miller, K. (2000). Routine hospital alcohol detoxification practice compared to symptom triggered management with an Objective Withdrawal Scale (CIWA-Ar). *American Journal on Addictions, 9* (2), 135–144.

Richter, K.P., Choi, W.S., McCool, R.M., Harris, K.J. & Ahluwalia, J.S. (2004). Smoking cessation services in U.S. methadone maintenance facilities. *Psychiatric Services, 55* (11), 1258–1264.

Richter, K.P., Gibson, C.A., Ahluwalia, J.S. & Schmelzle, K.H. (2001). Tobacco use and quit attempts among methadone maintenance clients. *American Journal of Public Health, 91* (2), 296–299.

Richter, K.P., McCool, R.M., Catley, D., Hall, M. & Ahluwalia, J.S. (2005). Dual pharmacotherapy and motivational interviewing for tobacco dependence among drug treatment patients. *Journal of Addictive Diseases, 24* (4), 79–90.

Rickels, K., Case, W.G., Schweizer, E., Garcia-Espana, F. & Fridman, R. (1990). Benzodiazepine dependence: Management of discontinuation. *Psychopharmacology Bulletin, 26* (1), 63–68.

Saunders, J.B., Aasland, O.G., Babor, T.F., de la Fuente, J.R. & Grant, M. (1993). Development of the Alcohol Use Disorders Identification Test (AUDIT): WHO collaborative project on early detection of persons with harmful alcohol consumption—II. *Addiction,* 88, 791–803.

Senft, R.A., Polen, M.R., Freeborn, D.K. & Hollis, J.F. (1997). Brief intervention in a primary care setting for hazardous drinkers. *American Journal of Preventive Medicine, 13* (6), 464–470.

Sims, T.H. & Fiore, M.C. (2002). Pharmacotherapy for treating tobacco dependence: What is the ideal duration of therapy? *CNS Drugs, 16* (10), 653–662.

Spiegel, D.A. (1999). Psychological strategies for discontinuing benzodiazepine treatment. *Journal of Clinical Psychopharmacology, 19, 6* (suppl. 2), 17s–22s.

Spiga, R., Huang, D.B., Meisch, R.A. & Grabowski, J. (2001). Human methadone self-administration: Effects of diazepam pretreatment. *Experimental and Clinical Psychopharmacology, 9* (1), 40–46.

Spiga, R., Martinetti, M.P., Meisch, R.A., Cowan, K. & Hursh, S. (2005). Methadone and nicotine self-administration in humans: A behavioral economic analysis. *Psychopharmacology (Berlin), 178* (2–3), 223–231.

Spiga, R., Schmitz, J. & Day, J. II. (1998). Effects of nicotine on methadone self-administration in humans. *Drug and Alcohol Dependence, 50* (2), 157–165.

Srivastava, A., Kahan, M. & Ross, S. (2007). The effect of methadone maintenance treatment on alcohol consumption: A systematic review. *Journal of Substance Abuse Treatment, 34* (2), 215–223.

Sullivan, J.T., Sykora, K., Schneiderman, J., Naranjo, C.A. & Sellers, E.M. (1989). Assessment of alcohol withdrawal: The revised Clinical Institute Withdrawal Assessment for Alcohol scale (CIWA-Ar). *British Journal of Addiction, 84* (11), 1353–1357.

Van Ameringen, M., Allgulander, C., Bandelow, B., Greist, J.H., Hollander, E., Montgomery, S.A. et al. (2003). WCA recommendations for the long-term treatment of social phobia. *CNS Spectrums, 8* (suppl. 1), 40–52.

Watson, S.J., Benson, J.A. Jr. & Joy, J.E. (2000). Marijuana and medicine—Assessing the science base: A summary of the 1999 Institute of Medicine report. *Archives of General Psychiatry, 57* (6), 547–552.

Wetterling, T., Kanitz, R.D., Rumpf, H.J., Hapke, U. & Fischer, D. (1998). Comparison of cage and mast with the alcohol markers CDT, gamma-GT, ALAT, ASAT and MCV. *Alcohol and Alcoholism, 33* (4), 424–430.

Zellweger, J.P. (2001). Anti-smoking therapies: Is harm reduction a viable alternative to smoking cessation? *Drugs, 61* (8), 1041–1044.

CHAPTER 12

Methadone and pain management

This chapter discusses management of both acute and chronic pain in MMT patients and provides some guidelines for physicians.

Acute pain

Patients on long-term MMT can develop analgesic tolerance to methadone, analgesic cross-tolerance to other opioids and hyperalgesia (lower pain threshold and heightened sensitivity to pain) from long-term opioid therapy (Alford et al., 2006; Doverty et al., 2001; Friedman et al., 2003). Therefore, when such patients are in acute pain, they derive little analgesic benefit from methadone and often require higher or more frequent opioid doses than other patient populations in order to obtain relief. There is minimal evidence to support the notion that treating pain with opioids will result in a relapse to opioid dependence (Alford et al., 2006). Indeed, some have argued that under-treatment of acute pain can cause relapse by encouraging the patient to self-medicate.

MANAGEMENT

The methadone-dispensing physician should address any patient concerns about pain management before prescribing opioids. Some patients will be concerned that any opioid use will trigger a relapse, while others might be afraid that their pain will be under-treated because of their addiction history. The physician should provide reassurance on both counts, explaining that short-term opioid use for pain is unlikely to trigger a relapse and that the patient's pain will be adequately treated. However, the physician should watch for any signs of relapse (e.g., continued requests for large doses of opioids long after the acute pain should have resolved, or refusal of consent to talk to the prescribing physician).

It is suggested that the physician start the patient at a dose that would normally be prescribed for a patient with a similar condition, and titrate upward if necessary. Non-opioid analgesics should be used concurrently. The opioid should be dispensed with the methadone (e.g., if the patient is on daily dispensing, the additional opioid should be dispensed daily as well). In the case of patients who were injection drug users, acetaminophen-opioid combinations are preferred because they are more difficult to inject. Opioids with a lower abuse liability (such as codeine and morphine) are preferred over those with greater liability (such as oxycodone or hydromorphone), and scheduled rather than as-needed dispensing is preferred for constant pain. Opioid agonist-antagonists such as pentazocine should be avoided.

Chronic pain

PREVALENCE

The prevalence of chronic pain within the MMT population appears to be higher than in the general population. A recent study of 170 MMT patients (Peles et al., 2005) found that about 55 per cent experienced chronic pain (defined as current pain lasting for six months or more) and had a significantly higher proportion of chronic illness (74.5 per cent) than patients without chronic pain (44.7 per cent). Of those with pain, only 13 per cent had mild pain, while the rest had moderate to very severe pain. Patients who had had pain for 10 or more years were those who had been prescribed the highest methadone dosage (182.1 +/– 59.2 mg/day). Therefore, the presence and duration of chronic pain seems to be correlated with methadone dose.

In another study, of 390 patients in MMT and 531 patients from short-term inpatient substance abuse treatment programs in New York State, the prevalence of chronic severe pain (defined as persistent pain for more than six months that is of moderate to severe intensity or that has significantly interfered with daily activities) was 37 per cent among MMT patients and 24 per cent among inpatients (Rosenblum et al., 2003). Pain in MMT patients was correlated with age, chronic illness, an ongoing, lifetime diagnosis of psychiatric illness, current psychiatric distress and duration of MMT treatment. This comorbidity also leads to increased use of health care services, and confirms the co-occurrence of severe medical and psychiatric problems with pain (Trafton et al., 2004).

MMT patients with pain will seek out opioid medications specifically in attempts to self-medicate while still demonstrating behaviours consistent with those of their peers without pain. Therefore, MMT programs need to have clear policies and screening procedures regarding chronic pain.

MANAGEMENT

There are no established guidelines for the use of other sustained-released opioids, such as MS Contin, for the management of chronic pain in MMT patients. It is important for physicians to approach chronic pain in this patient population within general chronic-pain guidelines (i.e., introduce a treatment agreement, monitor for compliance, and so on), keeping in mind that these patients are at higher risk for abuse and need closer monitoring. See the CPSO's *Evidence-Based Recommendations for Medical Management of Chronic Non-Malignant Pain* and *Methadone for Pain Guidelines.*

The physician should ensure, first of all, that the patient's methadone dose is adequate, and that the patient ingests it as prescribed at the same time every day.

After any organic pathology has been ruled out, the next step is to assess the nature of the pain (neuropathic vs. somatic), as well as the level of functional impairment that can be attributed to the pain alone. Consultation with a pain specialist is recommended.

In cases where the impairment is more attributable to active opioid dependence than to the pain itself, the patient should be encouraged to engage in intensive counselling, such as residential treatment and/or part-icipation in mutual aid groups.

The same pharmacy should be used for all prescriptions, and any pain medication prescribed for MMT patients should be dispensed along with the methadone. Short, frequent prescriptions are recommended. UDS results should be monitored to ensure they are consistent with the prescribed medication. If the patient is not responding to treatment or the urine drug screens reveal other substance use, the physician should re-evaluate the treatment plan.

References

Alford, D.P., Compton, P. & Samet, J. (2006). Acute pain management in patients receiving maintenance methadone or buprenorphine therapy. *Annals of Internal Medicine, 144,* 127–134.

Doverty, M., Somogyi, A.A., White, J.M., Bochner, F., Beare, C.H., Menelaou, A. et al., (2001). Methadone maintenance patients are cross-tolerant to the antinociceptive effects of morphine. *Pain, 93* (2), 155–163.

Friedman, R., Kamel, I., Perez, C. & Hamada, A. (2003). Severe intraoperative hypertension and opioid-resistant postoperative pain in a methadone-treated patient. *Journal of Pain, 4* (5), 289–290.

Peles, E., Schreiber, S., Gordon, J. & Adelson, M. (2005). Significantly higher methadone dose for methadone maintenance treatment (MMT) patients with chronic pain. *Pain, 113,* 340–346.

Rosenblum, A., Joseph, H., Fong, C., Kipnis, S., Cleland, C. & Portenoy, R.K. (2003). Prevalence and characteristics of chronic pain among chemically dependent patients in methadone maintenance and residential treatment facilities. *Journal of the American Medical Association, 289,* 237–238.

Trafton, J.A., Oliva, E.M., Horst, D.A., Minkel, J.D. & Humphreys, K. (2004). Treatment needs associated with pain in substance use disorder patients: Implications for concurrent treatment. *Drug and Alcohol Dependence, 73,* 23–31.

CHAPTER 13

MMT and concurrent psychiatric illness

This chapter provides information on concurrent psychiatric disorders, including prevalence rates and recommendations for screening and assessment of MMT patients for such disorders. This chapter also discusses treatment interventions, including pharmacotherapy.

Introduction to concurrent psychiatric disorders

PREVALENCE

Mental illness and addiction are chronic, remitting and relapsing conditions. Both are thought to arise from dysfunction in the limbic system and its projections. Moreover, both are caused by gene-environment interactions and are considered to be incurable diseases that are treatable, but progressive if left untreated. Both are major public health concerns that contribute significantly and cumulatively to death, disease and disability rates.

It is difficult to estimate the true prevalence of concurrent psychiatric and addictive disorders. There is little consistency in the use of objective diagnostic criteria in the settings in which these populations have been studied. In a report on one of the largest community-based samples, the Epidemiological Catchment Area Study (Regier et al., 1990), people with mental illness were demonstrated to have high lifetime prevalence rates of substance abuse. For example, the prevalence of addiction in patients with schizophrenia is estimated at 47 per cent, and up to 90 per cent of people with schizophrenia smoke regularly. There is clear cross-sectional evidence (Abbott et al., 1994; Brooner et al., 1997; Khantzian & Treece, 1985; Rounsaville et al., 1982; Chen et al., 1999; Strain et al., 1991) indicating a high range for lifetime prevalence (47 to 85 per cent) of a broad spectrum of psychiatric illnesses in people who have an opioid dependence, as compared to people who do not have substance dependencies.

Although people who have an opioid dependence show a higher prevalence of almost every major mental illness, the most common associations are with mood and anxiety disorders, eating disorders and personality disorders.

EXPLANATORY HYPOTHESES

There are several etiological explanations and popular hypotheses for the phenomenon of comorbidity, which are supported by varying levels of empirical evidence. Examples include:

- the self-medication hypothesis (patients use drugs to treat underlying emotional states and/or mental illness)
- the common factor model (a common factor, e.g., genetic or environmental, causes both mental illness and addiction)
- substance abuse models (mental health problems increase the chances of developing a substance use disorder)
- secondary psychopathology models (patients who use substances develop mental illness)
- bidirectional models (substance use and mental illness affect each other).

EFFECTS

The concurrence of mental illness and substance use has substantial social, economic and prognostic consequences. In general, such concurrent disorders have worse outcomes than does one or the other disorder alone. People with concurrent disorders also experience a higher rate of homelessness or unstable housing (Drake et al., 1991) and greater instability in social functioning (e.g., family conflict, financial difficulties and compromised social contact). There is evidence of earlier onset of mental illness (Noordsy et al., 1991) in people with substance use disorders, and a general exacerbation of mental health symptoms. Patients with concurrent disorders also experience more general health problems, are at greater risk of contracting HIV (Mahler, 1995) and have an increased risk of sexual and physical abuse (Bellack & Gearon, 1998).

Substance abuse (including tobacco addiction) complicates the management of psychiatric illness and negatively affects treatment retention and outcomes. In clinical settings, it is generally believed that the most common reason for relapse to mental illness is untreated substance abuse, and the most common cause of relapse to substance abuse is untreated mental illness.

Comorbidity poses significant challenges to patients, their families, the health care system and treatment providers. Some of the most salient issues include the difficulties involved in engaging those with a concurrent psychiatric disorder to accept treatment and to participate in appropriate integrated protocols to manage both disorders. Treatment adherence is a significant problem for people who have both a mental illness and addiction-related issues. Compromised treatment adherence, in turn, correlates with poorer treatment outcomes, increased hospitalization rates and increased levels of utilization of health and social services.

Screening for and assessment of concurrent disorders

It can be difficult to differentiate other psychiatric disorders from opioid-induced mental disorders and from the psychiatric symptoms that can be a feature of opioid abuse and dependence. These symptoms include intoxication, withdrawal, intoxication delirium, psychotic disorder (with onset during intoxication), mood disorders (with onset during intoxication), sexual dysfunction (with onset during intoxication) and sleep disorders (with onset either during intoxication or withdrawal) (APA, 2004).

Opioid-induced disorders are considered to be the direct consequence of the use of an opioid. They are generally expected to resolve once the opioid has reached levels below a certain threshold.

Assessment can be divided into six domains (NIDA, 1999):

1. psychiatric assessment and determination of the risk of harm to self or others
2. risk of intoxication and withdrawal
3. recovery environment
4. relapse risk
5. treatment acceptance or readiness to change
6. comprehensive medical assessment, including possible screening for pregnancy, sexually transmitted infections (STIs) and other communicable diseases.

Some of these domains fall outside the scope of this chapter.

The syndromes of intoxication and withdrawal can mimic or mask psychiatric syndromes and may also be a trigger for the development of psychiatric symptoms. One of the major challenges in clinical practice is to reach a reasonable level of diagnostic certainty when diagnosing a separate mental illness (as opposed to recognizing psychiatric symptoms) in individuals with an addiction. A psychiatric disorder is diagnosed if a person fulfils the required criteria from a list for a particular disorder in the DSM IV-TR (APA, 2004). More often than not, it is difficult to distinguish between a bona fide psychiatric illness and a substance-induced mental disorder, as the symptoms may be very similar.

Under ideal conditions, it is considered prudent, albeit impractical, to fully manage the withdrawal of a person and to allow three to four weeks of substance-free time before making an independent psychiatric diagnosis. In reality, however, the complexity of the diagnostic task often exceeds the available time and human resources available, especially when the patient has severe and persistent mental illness. In such situations, clinicians tend to rely on a combination of factors, such as information from collateral service providers and family members, the presence or absence of mental illness in the family history, the patient's clinical presentation during periods of abstinence or reduced use, and the temporal onset of the disorders (i.e., the answer to the question "Which came first—the addiction or the psychiatric symptoms?"). Even with these guidelines, it is often not possible to definitively and reliably diagnose independent psychiatric conditions in this population, and therefore the approach to the assessment and formulation of the diagnoses needs to be done in a longitudinal fashion.

Treating concurrent disorders

TREATMENT MODELS

There is evidence (Chi et al., 2006; Cacciola et al., 2001) that integrating treatment for addiction and mental illness yields better outcomes than providing it in a sequential fashion. In particular, a seamless treatment program provided by the same team allows for better outcomes than sequential, multiple treatments where the responsibility to navigate the system is often left up to the person with the concurrent disorders.

GENERAL PRINCIPLES

The overarching principle in managing patients with concurrent disorders is to treat the patient on the least restrictive level of care that is proven to be safe and likely to be effective. Under ideal circumstances the patient should be matched with the appropriate level of care (outpatient, residential or medically managed). Further, the principles of primary, secondary and tertiary prevention should be followed. This approach serves several important functions, such as preventing the development of substance abuse in persons with mental illness; avoiding seroconversion to HIV, hepatitis B or hepatitis C in patients who are opioid dependent and who are at risk; or optimizing rehabilitation efforts through multiple mechanisms.

Another general principle for treating concurrent disorders is to ensure the availability, accessibility and affordability of services. Ideally, treatment systems should also be flexible and comprehensive, and offer a continuum of services designed around the needs of the patient with concurrent disorders. One hallmark of individuals with mental illness and addiction is that relapse in one domain can trigger a relapse in the other—a fact that can place an additional burden on service providers.

STEP-BY-STEP RECOMMENDATIONS

The following steps are recommended for managing patients who present with concurrent psychiatric illness and opioid dependence.

Step 1: Assess for immediate risk of harm

The first priority in treatment is to ensure the patient's safety by conducting baseline and serial risk assessments. Patients who are considered to be at immediate and substantial risk of harm to themselves or others may need to be hospitalized, voluntarily or involuntarily. Admission to a psychiatric facility under the *Mental Health Act* is mandated if a person is suffering from a mental illness and is deemed to be at imminent and substantial risk of harming himself or herself. Once the patient is admitted, there is a further determination of the risk factors for intoxication or withdrawal, which are handled on their own merits.

The following questions (Sheehan et al., 1998) can help a clinician screen for suicidality and rate the risk of suicide:

- Have you ever made a suicide attempt?
- In the past month, did you:
  - think you'd be better off dead or wish you were dead?
  - want to harm yourself?
  - think about suicide?
  - have a suicide plan?
  - attempt suicide?

Note that most suicides happen when patients are intoxicated. A family history of suicide is also a risk factor.

Step 2: Distinguish between independent and substance-induced syndromes

As discussed above, if the psychiatric symptoms are considered to be substance induced (in the context of opioids, such symptoms can include intoxication, withdrawal, delirium, psychotic symptoms, mood symptoms, sexual dysfunction, sleep disorders, or any combination of these), it is considered reasonable to first have the person withdrawn from the substance prior to reassessing the patient for an independent psychiatric disorder. Alternative mechanisms to increase the validity of such diagnoses in non-ideal situations (such as looking at family history and presentation during abstinent periods) are described above. A patient may need to be placed in a withdrawal management program for this purpose, but this depends on the circumstances—in particular on whether the patient can reasonably be withdrawn safely in an ambulatory rather than a medical setting. Patients with severe mental illness can be socially, occupationally and/or residentially disenfranchised, and may therefore require admission to a residential or hospital setting for safe and effective withdrawal management.

Psychiatric rating scales as screening tools

The use of objective, quantifiable psychiatric rating scales ("clinimetrics") can enhance the sensitivity and specificity of a clinical screening process and help in monitoring progress and measuring treatment outcomes. These tools aid the clinician by providing a better understanding of the severity of the patient's psychiatric symptoms and are considered to be the standard of care when treating mental illness.

These psychiatric rating scales are designed to screen for specific symptoms and/or signs, and typically aim to cover the entire range of a particular disorder. Some of the tools are self-rating (score assigned by the patient), while others are completed by a physician or other health care provider. The level of complexity and the amount of training required to administer the scales vary from instrument to instrument. Two of these instruments, recommended for use in primary care settings to screen for the most salient psychiatric symptoms and disorders, are presented below. The challenge for physicians is to select an appropriate scale or set of scales for optimizing the assessment and management of patients in the particular treatment setting where the instrument(s) will be used.

One particularly useful screening tool is the Mini-International Neuro-Psychiatric Interview, or the MINI (Sheehan et al., 1998), which screens for 17 of the most commonly found psychiatric disorders in the DSM-IV. It is brief (takes about 15 minutes), highly sensitive and reliable, requires minimal training, and is compatible with use in primary care settings (although it is also useful in research). The MINI assists in the diagnoses of depression, anxiety disorders, psychotic disorders, substance use disorders and eating disorders, and also screens for suicidality. It has been translated into over 30 languages.

Depressive symptoms are among the most common psychiatric symptoms experienced by patients dealing with addiction. One scale useful in assessing and monitoring mood symptoms is the abbreviated Hamilton Depression Rating 7-Item Scale, or the HAM-7 (McIntyre et al., 2005). It is brief, practical and reliable, and has been validated in both primary care and mental health settings. The maximum score on this scale is 26; a score of less than 3 is consistent with a totally remitted mood state (euthymia). The standard of care is to work toward full remission (analagous to a blood pressure of 120/80). Further, the goal is also to achieve a return to previous (premorbid) levels of functioning if possible in all domains of the person's life, including socially, interpersonally and occupationally.

Tools such as these typically do not make the specific diagnosis of a mental disorder, but rather they screen for the symptoms associated with the particular disorder and allow clinicians to standardize patient care and treatment. Every assessment should also include a functional assessment, using all available sources of information about the patient's background, psychiatric history, physical health and safety, and previous psychiatric hospitalizations (if any), as well as an assessment of his or her relative strengths and functioning in occupational, social, academic and other domains.

Step 3: Integrate pharmacotherapy and psychotherapy or counselling

Note: Medication management for opioid dependence is discussed elsewhere in this manual. This section focuses on the salient aspects of pharmacotherapy for independent comorbid psychiatric disorders.

The goal of managing opioid dependence in people with a mental illness is to treat both disorders in an integrated fashion, strategically dovetailing psychosocial interventions with any applicable pharmacotherapy. It is generally not considered clinically useful to refer to either of the disease entities as "primary" or "secondary." It may be more prudent to consider both to be primary and to treat both disorders at the same time, especially if they both contribute to the patient's clinical presentation.

Clinicians should be cautious about using pharmacotherapy alone, and are advised instead to combine it routinely with psychosocial interventions to optimize outcomes. Medication should not be framed as the panacea for addiction, although medication may play an important role in its management. The treatment of addiction is a process, not an event. The medications used in the treatment of psychopathology are considered safe, not addictive, and do not cause euphoria.

Compliance issues can arise with patients who become involved with a 12-step facilitation group (TSF), such as Alcoholics Anonymous or Narcotics Anonymous, where they may in some cases encounter the dictum "a drug is a drug is a drug." Patients in such a situation need education in this regard. They should be encouraged to continue with their medication management, to discuss any issues with their care provider, and to not allow a sponsor or other group members to control their medication decisions.

Even if a patient is unable to maintain abstinence and sobriety from alcohol, tobacco or illicit drugs, the treatment of his or her independent psychiatric illness should nevertheless proceed, albeit with caution. The evidence indicates that even in the face of ongoing drug use, most medication forms for treating psychopathology are considered safe and effective—with a few exceptions, which are discussed under the subheading for the relevant disorder in the "Pharmacotherapy" section below.

Physicians of patients with concurrent disorders need to address the following questions regarding medication:

- Is this medication safe in overdose?
- What happens if this medication is combined with alcohol or other drugs?
- What is the abuse potential of the prescribed drug?
- What is the impact of non-adherence on the outcome?
- Is the medication still effective if the patient continues to use drugs or alcohol?

Step 4: Monitor and reassess during follow-up

Follow-up monitoring needs to be conducted in a longitudinal fashion. People with mental illness may progress more slowly through the stages of change, and there are vast interpersonal differences in the speed at which people recover from concurrent disorders. Typically, any treatment (whether outpatient or residential) lasting less than three months is of minimal value. The minimum time period for MMT is considered to be 12 months, and successful outcomes may require more than one treatment experience (NIDA, 1999). Care providers should, therefore, plan for a lengthy period of psychosocial rehabilitation and treatment, and should revisit the treatment plan and reassess the patient's motivation to change at least every six months.

PHARMACOTHERAPY

Bipolar mood disorder

Patients who have both bipolar mood disorder and a history of substance abuse tend to respond poorly to lithium carbonate (Nunes et al., 1990). Alternatives such as valproate and/or one of the atypical antipsychotic drugs (e.g., olanzapine, risperidone, quetiapine) may therefore be considered first-line treatment for this population with concurrent disorders. Carbamazepine or the newer anti-epileptic drugs may be considered for mood stabilization. Close monitoring of valproate, carbamazepine, or (if it is used) lithium levels is considered part of ongoing treatment management, as are serial liver function tests for the latter. Chronic use of alcohol and/or other medications can also lead to elevated liver functions, and alcohol consumption can lead to lithium toxicity. Early evidence shows that the use of quetiapine can decrease cravings in addicted bipolar patients (Brown et al., 2002). The use of carbamazepine (like that of alcohol) may, due to the induction of several liver enzymes, lower the blood levels of opioids and precipitate a withdrawal syndrome.

Depressive disorders

The goal of treating major depression and/or dysthymic disorder in people with opioid dependence is full remission of the depressive disorder as well as functional recovery as far as possible. Opioid-dependent patients with depressive symptoms often experience an improvement in these symptoms as a result of MMT alone (Petrakis et al., 1998). However, most of the clinical trials on opioid-dependent populations have included respondents who also used cocaine, thus complicating the translatability of the recommendations arising from these trials.

Treatment with a sedating antidepressant may interfere with sedating drugs like opioids, alcohol, barbiturates and benzodiazepines, and it may potentially cause life-threatening complications of psychomotor retardation. The first-line pharmacotherapy in this context is generally considered to be SNRIs (e.g., venlafaxine XR) or SSRIs (e.g., fluoxetine, paroxetine, citalopram, fluvoxamine or escitalopram), because of their high degree of efficacy, their tolerability and their safety profiles. Sertraline (Hamilton et al., 2000) tends to increase the levels of methadone in the initial stages, and fluvoxamine (DeMaria & Serota, 1999; Alderman & Frith, 1999) has been reported to display a pharmacokinetic drug interaction (CYP 3A4-mediated) with methadone; therefore, caution should be exercised if these are prescribed.

Some tricyclic antidepressants are considered to be effective, but their cardiotoxic effects are of concern—these medications can be lethal in overdose, and they also decrease the seizure threshold. For this reason, the tricyclics are usually best avoided in the opioid-dependent population. Bupropion may have the added advantage of optimizing the treatment of tobacco dependence in this population, which has high rates of such dependence. However, it should be prescribed with caution, especially with patients whose seizure threshold has been lowered by another drug or by a previous history of brain injury or seizures, or with patients who may be at risk of withdrawing from benzodiazepines, alcohol or barbiturates. Monoamine oxidase inhibitors (MAOIs) should also generally be avoided in this population.

When initiating antidepressant treatment, clinicians should be aware of the potential for risks of harm, especially in the early stages of treatment. Patients may require close observation. A safety contract and mobilization of support systems can be very helpful.

For the treatment of insomnia, non-benzodiazepine hypnotics are preferred. These include drugs like trazodone, zaleplon, zopiclone and quetiapine (the side-effects of which must be monitored), or tryptophan, which should be prescribed in combination with the implementation of sleep hygiene principles.

Psychotic disorders

Pharmacotherapy is the mainstay in managing psychotic disorders, as it is known to improve treatment retention. In this context of patients with substance abuse problems, the atypical antipsychotics have distinct advantages over the typical antipsychotics. In most situations today, the typical antipsychotics tend to be reserved for third-line use. The newer atypicals (e.g., clozapine, risperidone, olanzapine and quetiapine) have fewer extrapyramidal side-effects (with the exception of risperidone), target the most problematic symptoms of schizophrenia, have cognitive-enhancing qualities and have ultra-low risk of tardive dyskinesia. Tobacco consumption tends to also decrease when patients use atypical antipsychotics as compared to the older drug classes (George et al., 2000).

As the drugs in this class tend to be sedating, patients should be warned about potential psychomotor retardation effects when operating a vehicle or machinery. Clozapine likely has the most impact on reducing substance use, but is not indicated as a first-line antipsychotic due to the risk of agranulocytosis.

The antipsychotics are not considered to pose significant risk of pharmacokinetic interactions with methadone, but the issues of weight gain and diabetogenic potential need to be closely monitored.

Personality disorders

No pharmacotherapy is currently registered or indicated for use in this category—the mainstay of treatment is psychosocial in nature. The high level of comorbid antisocial personality disorder in the population of patients on MMT is of concern, and this disorder may not be amenable to treatment with medication. However, antisocial behaviours such as crime may be reduced once the patient is stabilized on methadone. When making a diagnosis, the physician should be sure to consider any childhood history of conduct disorder and any antisocial behaviour that predates drug use. Borderline personality disorder should be managed with dialectical behavioural therapy if it is available, or with appropriate motivational interviewing techniques and behavioural interventions such as contingency management.

Attention-deficit/hyperactivity disorder (ADHD)

Patients with a history of substance abuse who are prescribed dextroamphetamine or methylphenidate may be at increased risk of abusing these drugs. The use of modafinil has not been tested in the substance-dependent population, and neither has the use of atomoxetine. Both, however, may hold promise for management of ADHD in people with a history of substance dependence, as these drugs hold low abuse and diversion risks. Bupropion may be used as a second-line agent with no abuse liability.

Anxiety disorders

These include generalized anxiety disorder, panic disorder, agoraphobia, social anxiety disorder, specific phobias and posttraumatic stress disorder.

Both SNRIs (e.g., venlafaxine XR) and SSRIs (with the possible exceptions of sertraline and fluvoxamine) may be considered useful. Most of the same principles for treating depressive disorders in the opioid-dependent population also apply to the treatment of anxiety disorders in this context. However, with anxiety disorders, the general approach is to "start low and go slow." The time from initiation of treatment to response may be longer than with depression.

It should be noted that bupropion is considered to be stimulating and can exacerbate anxiety symptoms in sensitive individuals.

Fatal interactions can occur when combining benzodiazepines with methadone or other opioids, with or without the concomitant use of alcohol. Benzodiazepines further have an established abuse risk and can be disinhibiting in some subpopulations, especially when combined with alcohol. They may also pose a diversion risk. It is thus recommended that benzodiazepines be avoided for patients on MMT other than in exceptional cases where the potential benefits clearly outweigh the risks.

Eating disorders

No pharmacotherapeutic trials specifically guide the treatment of eating disorders (such as anorexia nervosa and bulimia nervosa) in the opioid-dependent population. SSRIs and psychosocial interventions are considered the mainstay.

Regarding drug interactions, the principles outlined in the discussion of anxiety disorders above may apply, but higher doses of SNRIs may be required in the case of eating disorders. The use of bupropion is best avoided in this population due to the potential seizure risk in patients who have electrolyte imbalances resulting from purging or starvation.

PSYCHOSOCIAL INTERVENTIONS

A wide variety of psychotherapeutic modalities and approaches have been proven to be helpful in managing patients with concurrent disorders. Many foundational mental health services have been adapted to meet the needs of this population, including stage-wise interventions (engagement, persuasion, active treatment, relapse prevention):

- case management
- family network therapy
- psychoeducation
- housing assistance
- involuntary interventions
- social skills training
- vocational rehabilitation
- training in illness management skills
- crisis response services
- assertive community treatment
- enhanced inpatient services
- motivational interviewing
- cognitive-behavioural therapy
- relapse prevention programs
- 12-step facilitation (e.g., Dual Recovery Anonymous [DRA], sometimes known as "double trouble groups").

Note that people with mental illness may at times have difficulty finding an appropriate 12-step group, and may require assistance finding one with a philosophy that allows for maintenance treatment with methadone or other pharmacotherapeutic interventions.

Caregivers working with this population need to pay special attention to maintaining optimal treatment adherence, which is usually accomplished by using a cognitive-behavioural model and principles of motivational enhancement therapy. The following approaches can also help in this regard:

- simplifying medication regimes (e.g., favouring once-a-day dosing over multiple doses per day)
- psychoeducation (to inform the patient of the expected benefits and potential side-effects of medication)
- communicating the expected duration of treatment
- mobilizing support from significant others
- using depot formulations if available
- integrating the treatment regime into a patient's daily routine.

Overcoming challenges

The psychiatric assessment and management of patients with concurrent disorders can be particularly challenging. Common obstacles include (Mueser et al., 2003):

- on the part of the clinician:
  - failure to take a proper history
  - excessive attention to the primary-secondary distinction.
- on the part of the patient:
  - denial and minization
  - confusion about the effects of substance use.

People with severe mental illness and addiction issues may experience significant cognitive deficits, and hence find it difficult to progress in a treatment system that relies on the patient's cognitive abilities to move through the stages of change. There is also often a further barrier of financial constraints, as many people with severe mental illness have limited incomes. Finally, those who are in the precontemplation stage, or who are otherwise not ready to enter treatment, may be prone to develop further complications of concurrent disorders while they remain untreated.

Summary

The established high prevalence rates of psychopathology in patients with opioid dependence and those in MMT pose significant challenges and demand special skills from physicians who prescribe methadone. The high prevalence of tobacco use and the increased risk of contracting communicable diseases among this population also call for special approaches to optimize outcomes. Multimodal longitudinal treatment that integrates psychosocial interventions and pharmacotherapy is considered the standard of treatment, with close monitoring of any safety concerns. Ideally, a patient in this population should be managed with the least restrictive level of care that is appropriate.

Only limited empirical evidence exists to guide MMT practices with the mentally ill population. Because comorbid psychiatric and medical illnesses can complicate a maintenance regime and decrease compliance, they may need to be managed aggressively. A pragmatic approach and integrated management of the two conditions are considered the standard of care to ensure optimal outcomes for both spectra of disorders. Treatment should be conducted according to a "time unlimited" treatment paradigm, where both disorders are treated at the same time, albeit in a longitudinal fashion, by the same team of health care providers.

References

Abbott, P.J., Weller, S.B. & Walker, S.R. (1994). Psychiatric disorders of opioid addicts entering treatment: Preliminary data. *Journal of Addictive Diseases, 13*, 1–11.

Alderman, C.P. & Frith, P.A. (1999). Fluvoxamine-methadone interaction. *Australian and New Zealand Journal of Psychiatry, 33*, 99–101.

American Psychiatric Association (APA). (2004). *Diagnostic and Statistical Manual of Mental Disorders* (4th ed., text revision). Washington, DC: Author.

Bellack, A.S. & Gearon, J.S. (1998). Substance abuse treatment for people with schizophrenia. *Addictive Behaviours, 23*, 749–766.

Brooner, R.K., King, V.L., Kidorf, M., Schmidt, C.W. Jr. & Bigelow, G.E. (1997). Psychiatric and substance use comorbidity among treatment-seeking opioid abusers. *Archives of General Psychiatry, 54* (1), 71–80.

Brown, E.S., Netjek, V.A., Perantie, D.C. & Bobadilla, L, (2002). Quetiapine in bipolar disorder and cocaine dependence. *Bipolar Disorders, 4*, 406–411.

Cacciola, J.S., Alterman, A.I., Rutherford, M.J., McKay, J.R. & Mulvaney, F.D. (2001). The relationship of psychiatric comorbidity to treatment outcomes in methadone maintained patients. *Drug and Alcohol Dependence, 61* (3), 271–280.

Chen, C.C., Tsai, S.Y., Su, L.W., Yang, T.W., Tsai, C.J. & Hwu, H.G. (1999). Psychiatric co-morbidity among male heroin addicts: Differences between hospital and incarcerated subjects in Taiwan. *Addiction, 94*, 825–832.

Chi, F.W., Satre, D.D. & Weisner, C. (2006). Chemical dependency patients with cooccurring psychiatric diagnoses: Service patterns and 1-year outcomes. *Alcoholism, Clinical and Experimental Research, 30* (5), 851–859.

DeMaria, P.A. & Serota, R.D. (1999). A therapeutic use of the methadone fluvoxamine drug interaction. *Journal of Addictive Diseases, 18*, 5–12.

Drake, R.E., Osher, F.C. & Wallach, M.A. (1991). Homelessness and dual diagnosis. *American Psychologist, 46*, 1149–1158.

George, T.P., Ziedonis, D.M., Feingold, A., Pepper, W.T., Satterburg, C.A., Winkel, J. et al. (2000). Nicotine transdermal patch and atypical antipsychotic medications for smoking cessation in schizophrenia. *American Journal of Psychiatry, 157*, 1835–1842.

Hamilton, S.P., Nunes, E.V., Janal, M. & Weber, L. (2000). The effect of sertraline on methadone plasma levels in methadone maintained patients. *American Journal on Addictions 9*, 63–69.

Khantzian, E.J. & Treece, C. (1985). DSM-III psychiatric diagnosis of narcotic addicts. Recent findings. *Archives of General Psychiatry, 4*, 1067–1071.

Mahler, J.C. (1995). HIV, substance abuse, and mental illness. In Lehman, A.F. & Dixon, L.B. (Eds.), *Double Jeopardy, Chronic Mental Illness and Substance Use Disorders.* Langhorne, PA: Harwood Academic Publishers.

McIntyre, R.S., Konarski, J.Z., Mancini, D.A., Fulton, K.A., Parikh, S.V., Grigoriadis, S. et al. (2005). Measuring the severity of depression and remission in primary care: Validation of the HAMD-7 scale. *Canadian Medical Association Journal, 173*, 1327–1334.

Mueser, K.T., Noordsy, D.L., Drake, R.E. & Fox, L. (Eds.). (2003). *Integrated Treatment for Dual Disorders.* New York: Guilford Press.

National Institute of Health, National Institute of Addiction (NIDA). (1999). *Principles of Drug Addiction Treatment: A Research-Based Guide.* Available: www.drugabuse.gov/PODAT/PODATIndex.html.

Noordsy, D.L., Drake, R.E., Teague, G.B., Osher, F.C., Hurlbut, C., Beaudett, M.S. et al. (1991). Subjective experiences related to alcohol use among schizophrenics. *Journal of Nervous and Mental Diseases, 179*, 410–414.

Nunes, E.V., McGrath, P.J., Wager, S. & Quitkin, F.M. (1990). Lithium treatment for cocaine abusers with bipolar spectrum disorders. *American Journal of Psychiatry, 147* (5), 655–657.

Petrakis, I., Carroll, K.M., Nich, C., Gordon, L., Kosten, T. & Rounsaville, B. (1998). Fluoxetine treatment of depressive disorders in methadone maintained opioid addicts. *Drug and Alcohol Dependence, 50*, 221–226.

Regier, D.A., Farmer, M.E., Rae, D.S., Locke, B.Z., Keith, S.J., Judd, L.L. et al. (1990). Comorbidity of mental disorders with alcohol and other drug abuse: Results from the Epidemiological Catchment Area study. *Journal of the American Medical Association, 264*, 2511–2518.

Rounsaville, B.J., Weissman, M.M., Kleber, H. & Wilber, C. (1982). Heterogeneity of psychiatric diagnosis in treated opiate addicts. *Archives of General Psychiatry, 39*, 161–168.

Sheehan, D.V., Lecrubier, Y., Sheehan, K.H., Amorim, P., Janavs, J., Weiller, E. et al. (1998). The Mini International Neuropsychiatric Interview (MINI): The development and validation of a structured diagnostic psychiatric interview for DSM-IV and ICD-10. *Journal of Clinical Psychiatry, 59*, 22–33.

Strain, E.C. (2002). Assessment and treatment of comorbid psychiatric disorders in opioid-dependent patients. *Clinical Journal of Pain, 18*, s14–s27.

Strain, E.C., Brooner, R.K. & Bigelow, G.E. (1991). Clustering of multiple substance use and psychiatric diagnoses in opiate addicts. *Drug and Alcohol Dependence, 27*, 127–134.

CHAPTER 14

MMT and concurrent medical disorders

This chapter discusses the interaction of MMT and concurrent, ongoing medical conditions. In particular, it discusses HIV and HCV, two infectious conditions that are especially prevalent among the opioid-using population. The sections on each of these two viruses cover prevalence, screening methods and clinical management approaches for MMT patients who also have the conditions. The chapter concludes with a brief discussion of how several other ongoing conditions can affect MMT.

HIV

PREVALENCE

Injection drug use, including the injection of opioids, is one of the leading risk factors for acquiring HIV (human immunodeficiency virus) infection. Recent data shows that 19.6 per cent of new positive HIV tests in Canada result from such use (Public Health Agency of Canada, 2005). Of women who tested positive for HIV in the first half of 2005, 38 per cent used injection drugs (Public Health Agency of Canada, 2005). The prevalence of HIV infection among such users has been estimated to be 5.1 per cent in Toronto (Research Group on Drug Use, 2004), and as high as 14.7 per cent in certain regions of Ontario (Millson et al., 2003). In Vancouver, it has been found to be even higher—23 per cent (Strathdee, 1997)—though some say the rate of new HIV infections in that city is decreasing among people who use injection drugs (Anderson, 2000).

The relatively high prevalence of HIV in this population can be explained by the risky behaviours associated with injecting drugs. For example, in one study, 27.6 per cent of people who use injection drugs, including 20.2 per cent of those who were HIV-positive, reported having shared needles in the past six months (Wood et al., 2001). Unsafe sexual practices are also highly prevalent in this population (Tyndall et al., 2002). In one study, 4.8 per cent of people who were HIV-negative and who used injection drugs had an HIV-positive sexual partner at the time of the study (Kerr et al., 2006). An important consideration is that 40 per cent of people who use drugs are in a sexual relationship with a non-user. These non-using partners are often women of childbearing age (Health Canada, 2001).

MMT has been shown to reduce HIV risk-taking behaviour (Gowing et al., 2004) and thus can reduce the rate of new HIV infections and the transmission of HIV (Mattick et al., 2003).

SCREENING AND ASSESSMENT

Patients who are HIV-negative or have unknown HIV status

The CPSO *Methadone Maintenance Guidelines* recommend that patients who present for methadone maintenance treatment (MMT) undergo HIV testing. Patients should provide informed consent for this test, following adequate pre-test counselling (Tessier et al., 2001). This counselling should include:

- assessing individual risk factors for HIV infection (e.g., injection drug use with needle sharing, unsafe sexual practices)
- explaining the HIV test itself (see below)
- clarifying the difference between HIV infection and AIDS
- inquiring into the patient's support systems

- informing the patient that HIV infection is reportable to the department of public health (depending on the jurisdiction).

Because of the reportability of a positive HIV test, some patients may prefer to have their HIV tests performed anonymously. Most provinces permit certain sites to perform anonymous HIV testing.

Patients who are being considered for HIV testing should be informed that the test checks a blood sample for antibodies produced by the body in response to HIV infection (TPH). The body can take up to 12 weeks to generate these antibodies after an infection takes place (the "window period"), so an HIV test performed within 12 weeks of a potential exposure may be falsely negative—patients must therefore be retested 12 weeks after their most recent high-risk exposure.

The initial HIV test is an ELISA (enzyme-linked immunosorbent assay). All positive ELISA tests are confirmed with a more reliable test called a Western Blot, which is very specific for HIV infection. Some HIV rapid tests are becoming available, though none are in widespread use.

If a patient claims to have had, within the past 72 hours, high-risk exposure (i.e., unprotected sex or needle sharing) to someone who is HIV-positive or at very high risk of being HIV-positive, the physician should consider offering ARV (antiretroviral) PEP (post-exposure prophylaxis), which can help prevent HIV infection after such an exposure (Tessier et al., 2001). The local department of public health or a physician knowledgeable in HIV should be consulted prior to initiating ARV PEP.

If the patient's HIV test comes back negative, he or she should be offered post-test counselling (Tessier et al., 2001). During this counselling session, the patient should be reminded about the window period and advised to seek another test three months after the most recent potential exposure to HIV. The counselling session should also be used to reinforce safer sex practices and safer needle use. Information about needle exchange programs can be obtained from the local public health department.

An "indeterminate" HIV test result should be discussed with the testing laboratory as well as with a physician knowledgeable in HIV or the local public health department.

Patients who are HIV-positive

If the patient's HIV test comes back positive, the patient should be informed that he or she has been infected with the HIV virus and that it can be transmitted to others. Again, safer sex and safer needle use should be discussed and encouraged. The patient should be encouraged to speak with a supportive, trusted person about the result. If such a person does not exist, the patient can contact an AIDS information line[1] for support and information about other resources. Patients will eventually have to notify their recent sexual partner(s) about their HIV seroconversion so that the partner(s) can also be tested for HIV. All patients who test positive for HIV should be referred immediately to a physician knowledgeable in HIV.

Assessing an HIV-positive patient for MMT requires the collection of a complete medical history. In particular, the patient should be asked:

- When did you first test positive for HIV?
- Do you know when you may have seroconverted with HIV (i.e., experienced an unexplained flu-like illness)?
- Have you had any chronic symptoms from the HIV infection (e.g., wasting, fatigue, diarrhea, peripheral neuropathy)?
- Have you had any complications from the HIV infection? Complications can include oral or esophageal candidiasis, pneumocystis carinii (PCP), pneumonia, cerebral toxoplasmosis, cryptococcal meningitis, tuberculosis (either latent or active infection), M. avium complex (MAC infection), cytomegalovirus (CMV) infection, lymphoma, cervical cancer, Kaposi's sarcoma and so forth.
- What antiretroviral medications are you on? Have you been adhering to your treatment regimen?
- Have you experienced any side-effects from your medication? Have you had other ARV treatment regimens in the past? If so, why were they discontinued?

It may also be useful to know the patient's most recent CD4 and viral load counts, as well as the lowest that the CD4 count has fallen in the past.

1 Contact Toronto Public Health's AIDS & Sexual Health InfoLine at 416 392-2437 (outside Toronto 1 800 668-2437).

A PPD skin test history should be obtained, and so should a complete vaccination history. Pneumococcal, influenza, tetanus-diptheria (with or without polio), and hepatitis A and/or B vaccines should all be considered in HIV-positive patients. Any additional past medical history (such as hepatitis C co-infection) and psychiatric history are also important. Finally, a social history is critical for HIV-positive patients in order to assess their sexual activity, level of functioning and support systems.

If the patient already has a regular primary care physician who manages his or her HIV infection, there is not much more for the methadone provider to do with respect to the HIV other than, if it seems appropriate, obtaining written consent from the patient to communicate with the HIV physician and to acquire a copy of the positive HIV test result and any other relevant medical records. An HIV-positive patient who does not have regular follow-up for the HIV infection should be referred to a physician knowledgeable in HIV without delay.

TREATING HIV PATIENTS IN MMT

MMT and ARV therapy

People who inject drugs are less likely than other HIV risk groups to receive ARV therapy (Clarke et al., 2003). MMT has been shown to improve adherence to ARVS among this population (Wood et al., 2005), resulting in better clinical outcomes (Antela, 2001). Indeed, treatment of a substance use disorder is often a prerequisite for successful ARV therapy (Dybul, 2002). Since HIV treatment guidelines are constantly changing, ARV therapy should be initiated and monitored by a physician knowledgeable in HIV (Dybul, 2002; Yeni et al., 2004).

A very important consideration for any methadone-prescribing physician is the potential for drug interactions between methadone and several of the available ARV medications. Methadone is metabolized via the hepatic P450 system, in particular the enzymes 3A4, 2B6 and 2D622. Several antiretroviral medications also interact with these P450 pathways (Clarke et al., 2003; Dybul, 2002). These drug interactions could potentially, though not necessarily, result in increased or decreased levels of either methadone or the ARVS. It is important to be aware that P450 inducers and inhibitors can affect methadone metabolism both when they are started and when they are stopped.

The type and degree of possible interaction varies depending on the specific ARV medication involved. NRTIS (nucleoside reverse transcriptase inhibitors) do not have a clinically significant effect on methadone metabolism; however, methadone may increase levels of AZT (zidovudine) and may decrease levels of d4T (stavudine) and the non-EC formulation of DDI (didanosine). The NNRTIS (non-nucleoside reverse transcriptase inhibitors) efavirenz and nevirapine are 3A4 inducers and can decrease methadone levels. This interaction may result in the onset of opioid withdrawal symptoms and a need to increase the dose of methadone by 5 to 10 mg per day after seven days of NNRTI therapy. The PIs (protease inhibitors) have generally been considered 3A4 and 2D6 inhibitors (Donaher et al., 2006), which means that in theory they could result in increased levels of methadone; however, according to several sources (Dybul, 2002; Addiction Treatment Forum, 2005), the PIs amprenavir, nelfinavir and lopinavir actually appear to *decrease* methadone levels, potentially causing opioid withdrawal symptoms. There is no known interaction between atazanavir and methadone. Methadone may decrease levels of the PI amprenavir.

Prior to initiating MMT for any HIV-positive patient who is receiving ARV medications, the methadone-prescribing physician should contact the patient's HIV physician to discuss any suggestions he or she may have regarding adjustments to the ARV regimen or to the monitoring of its efficacy and/or toxicity. Similarly, an HIV-positive methadone patient should notify the methadone prescriber in advance if he or she is going to start ARVS so the physician can plan for any potential methadone dose adjustments. It is good practice to educate patients about possible drug interactions, to monitor them closely and to adjust the methadone dose if necessary based on each patient's response to the new drug. This approach is preferable to adjusting the dose of methadone in anticipation of an interaction (Addiction Treatment Forum, 2005).

Additional useful resources on methadone drug interactions can be found at www.drug-interactions.com and www.atforum.com.

SUMMARY

People who are opioid dependent and use injection drugs—and their partners—are at increased risk for HIV infection. MMT can reduce risky drug-taking behaviour and, as a result, can reduce the risk of HIV transmission. Guidelines advise testing all new methadone maintenance clients for HIV.

Doctors who prescribe methadone are in a unique position of seeing HIV-positive patients who are often otherwise lost to follow-up. Because of the potential for clinical improvement of a patient's HIV condition, as well as the potential benefit of reducing HIV transmission to others, it has been argued that appropriate opioid-dependent, HIV-positive patients should be "fast-tracked" into MMT where possible (March, 2000).

Hepatitis C

PREVALENCE AND EFFECTS

Hepatitis C virus (HCV) is a single-stranded RNA virus that belongs to the flaviviridae family. This virus is constantly mutating, allowing it to evade a patient's immune system (Canadian Liver Foundation, 2000). While three per cent of the world's population is infected with HCV (Zou et al., 2000; Sherman et al., 2007), 0.8 to one per cent of the Canadian population has been diagnosed with hepatitis C. Currently 250,000 Canadians are living with HCV infection, and 5,000 new cases are diagnosed nationwide each year (Wong & Lee, 2006).

There are six genotypes of HCV, which are distributed geographically as follows: genotypes 1 to 3 are found worldwide, genotypes 4 and 5 in Africa and genotype 6 in Asia (Zou et al., 2000). In Canada, genotypes 1 to 3 are prevalent, with genotype 1 being the most common (Andonov & Chaudhary, 1994).

HCV is spread through blood or other body fluids that are contaminated with the virus (Wong & Lee, 2006; Sherman et al., 2007). There are several risk factors, but the most important is injection drug use, which accounts for the majority (approximately 60 per cent) of HCV cases in Canada. Even a single episode of injection drug use in the remote past is sufficient for HCV transmission. Approximately 90 per cent of people who use injection drugs acquire HCV within the first year of using drugs.

Travel or residence in endemic regions such as Egypt (where 15 to 20 per cent of the population is infected), Pakistan (where 10 per cent of the population is infected), and parts of Asia (e.g., Vietnam) is the second most common risk factor (Sherman et al. 2007; Wong & Lee 2006).

Blood products and organ transplantation prior to 1990 are also risk factors and account for 13 per cent of HCV cases (Sherman et al., 2007; Wong & Lee, 2006). Current practices in Canada have reduced the risk of HCV infection from blood transfusion to less than one in every 3,000,000 units transfused (Wong & Lee, 2006). Needle-stick injuries are associated with some risk (about one to three per cent risk of HCV seroconversion). Sharing contaminated intranasal cocaine equipment (e.g., straw or rolled-up money) is becoming associated with HCV infection. Body piercing and tattooing have also been reported as potential modes of HCV transmission.

Sexual transmission among long-term sexual partners with continuing sexual exposure and no other risk factors is low (less than five per cent). Casual contact such as shaking hands, kissing or sharing eating utensils does *not* transmit HCV.

The risk of vertical transmission (mother to newborn) is approximately four to seven per cent and rises with HIV co-infection and high maternal HCV viral load (Canadian Paediatric Society, 2008). Breastfeeding does not change the risk of HCV infection in the neonate, nor does the route of delivery (vaginal versus caesarian section).

NATURAL HISTORY

The mean incubation period for HCV is six to eight weeks. Acute infection with HCV is typically asymptomatic (in 60 to 75 per cent of cases), or may present with only mild flu-like symptoms with little or no jaundice (Wong & Lee, 2006; Hoofnagle, 1997). Another 20 to 30 per cent of patients with acute infection present with symptoms such as malaise, fatigue, lethargy, anorexia, abdominal pain, arthralgias, jaundice, mild hepatosplenomegaly and maculopapular rash, lasting two to 12 weeks. Of patients who have had acute infections, 15 to 50 per cent spontaneously clear the infection, whereas 50 to 85 per cent continue with chronic infection. HCV clearance occurs in most cases within 12 weeks (Sherman et al., 2007).

Chronic infection is generally asymptomatic but can also be characterized by malaise, nausea, abdominal pain and pruritus, associated with fluctuating alanine transaminase (ALT) levels (Wong & Lee, 2006). Serious complications of HCV occur a few decades after initial infection. About 20 to 30 years after acute infection, the risk of cirrhosis is about 20 per cent. After cirrhosis has developed, the risk of hepatocellular carcinoma (HCC) is one to four per cent per year (Seeff, 1997). In those who develop cirrhosis, the survival rate is 80 per cent at 10 years with a potential risk of decompensation (ascites, jaundice, variceal hemorrhage or hepatic encephalopathy). HCV remains the leading indication for liver transplantation in North America.

Extrahepatic manifestations of HCV may include mixed essential cryoglobulinemia, membranous or membranoproliferative glomerulonephritis, non-Hodgkin's lymphoma, Sjogren's syndrome, lichen planus and porphyria cutanea tarda (Wong & Lee, 2006).

Prognostic factors affecting the rate of progression to cirrhosis include sex (men progress more quickly than women), older age at infection acquisition (those over 40 years old progress faster), longer duration of infection, immune suppression (e.g., HIV co-infection), chronic hepatitis B co-infection, moderate or heavy alcohol use (more than 50 g of alcohol daily increases the speed of progression) and weight issues (obesity speeds progression) (Wong & Lee, 2006). In addition, prognosis is also related to hepatic pathology, such as the type and amount of liver inflammation and fibrosis (which can be determined through a liver biopsy) (Alberti et al., 2002).

SCREENING AND IDENTIFICATION

Acute vs. chronic infection

Screening for HCV infection should consist of serological testing for antibodies against HCV (anti-HCV) (Pawlotsky, 2002; Sherman et al., 2007). Testing is indicated for patients with risk factors for HCV and those with abnormal aminotransferase levels (Sherman et al., 2004; Alter et al., 2003; NIH, 2002). A positive anti-HCV result cannot distinguish between acute and chronic HCV infection, since antibodies may persist throughout a person's life. Chronic infection can be confirmed with qualitative HCV RNA testing.

Patients who have normal ALT levels and test positive for anti-HCV may have spontaneously cleared an HCV infection in the past, and further testing is required for diagnostic purposes. However, patients who have abnormal ALT levels and test positive for anti-HCV are usually diagnosed with chronic HCV infection (Wong & Lee, 2006). For these patients, further testing with HCV RNA may not be necessary to confirm chronic HCV status.

In the presence of normal ALT levels, chronic HCV can be confirmed by ordering qualitative HCV RNA testing (Pawlotsky, 2002; Hino et al., 1994). A positive HCV RNA result indicates active HCV replication and is consistent with chronic HCV.

In the case of acute infection, HCV RNA disappears when the infection resolves, whereas, in chronic infection, HCV RNA levels are stable over time. Therefore, a single negative qualitative HCV RNA test may be due to fluctuating virus levels or degradation of HCV RNA after sampling, or it may mean that a previous HCV infection has been cleared. Thus, a negative test result should be repeated six months later to distinguish patients with spontaneously resolving HCV infection from chronic carriers.

Newborn screening

The optimal method and timing of testing newborns of HCV-positive mothers is unknown. The prevalence of HCV in pregnancy is approximately one to two per cent (Zarski & Leroy, 1999). Antibodies to HCV are passively transferred in utero and are detectable for more than a year after delivery (Pawlotsky, 2002). HCV RNA levels decline if the infection has cleared. Infants can undergo anti-HCV testing after 12 months of age, or qualitative HCV RNA testing at six to 12 months (or later if anti-HCV is positive).

PREVENTIVE MEASURES

Educating high-risk substance users about primary and secondary prevention should be an integral part of all health care visits. People who use injection drugs should be educated about safer injection practices, such as avoiding sharing of injection equipment with others and using new syringes for each injection (Edlin et al., 2005). Access to HCV treatment requires treatment of substance use disorders; for example, offering MMT to patients with opioid dependence provides an opportunity to be considered for treatment (Edlin et al., 2005).

Secondary prevention measures include counselling about the transmission of HCV to other individuals and about progression of liver disease. HCV transmission among household contacts has not been demonstrated (Zarski & Leroy, 1999). The following prevention measures, however, should be adopted by those sharing a household with patients who are HCV-positive:

- Avoid sharing sharp items contaminated with blood (e.g., razors, nail clippers, toothbrushes).
- Cover up open wounds.
- Dispose of used needles and sharp instruments using universal precautions.
- Inform sexual partners and practise safe sex.

HCV-positive patients should also refrain from donating blood, organs, tissues and sperm.

Patients with HCV should follow precautions to decrease the likelihood that the disease will progress. Losing weight is recommended for obese patients and abstaining from alcohol use is recommended (Zarski & Leroy, 1999), since heavy alcohol intake has been shown to accelerate the progression of liver disease and increase the risk of HCC. Patients should be vaccinated against hepatitis A and B in order to avoid co-infection, and screening for HIV is also recommended because those who are co-infected are at higher risk of progression to cirrhosis (Edlin et al., 2005).

TREATING HCV PATIENTS

Acute HCV infection

Early treatment of acute HCV infection has been shown to be effective at preventing the development of chronic infection (Wiegand et al., 2006). The decision to begin treatment should be based on the presence of icteric hepatitis, which is a good prognostic indicator of HCV clearance. Treatment of acute HCV infection should be delayed in patients with icteric hepatitis, since 40 to 50 per cent of this population clears the virus spontaneously within 12 weeks (Gerlach et al., 2003; Jauncey et al., 2004). If HCV RNA persists after 12 weeks, treatment should be initiated, which will lead to viral clearance 80 per cent of the time (Sherman et al., 2007). Asymptomatic patients, especially those with non-icteric hepatitis, are less likely to clear the virus spontaneously, and should be considered for earlier treatment after diagnosis. Recent trials have demonstrated a greater than 90 per cent sustained response rate in terms of achieving undetectable HCV RNA with the administration of pegylated interferon alfa-2b for up to 24 weeks, depending on the genotype (Jaeckel et al., 2001; Wiegand et al., 2006; Kamal et al., 2006).

Chronic HCV infection

The decision to treat patients with chronic HCV depends on many factors, including the patient's risk of disease progression, likelihood of response, presence of comorbid conditions and patient choice. A full evaluation to assess for signs of liver disease and contraindications for antiviral therapy should be completed prior to making a final decision. Clinical assessment should include inquiries about past and current medical conditions such as cardiac and renal disease, seizures, substance use disorders, seizure disorders, psychiatric disorders, autoimmune diseases and the presence of HIV or hepatitis B co-infection. Laboratory assessment should include complete blood count, PT, INR, albumin, AST, ALT, bilirubin, ALP, HbsAg, HIV, TSH, ANA, glucose, creatinine, serum beta-hCG (to exclude pregnancy) and urinalysis (Wong & Lee, 2006; Sherman et al., 2004). Further investigations may include an electrocardiogram for patients older than 50 years or those with a history of coronary heart disease, and fundoscopic examination for patients older than 50 years with a history of high blood pressure or diabetes mellitus (Sherman et al., 2007).

ALT levels alone should not determine whether to proceed with treatment. Approximately 30 per cent of patients with chronic HCV have normal ALT levels (Bacon, 2002). Most of these patients have mild or no inflammation and fibrosis, and the rate of disease progression is less than that of patients with elevated ALT levels (Mathurin et al., 1998). Some chronic HCV patients, however, have advanced fibrosis and cirrhosis on liver biopsy. Response to treatment among patients with normal ALT levels has been similar to that of patients with abnormal levels (Shiffman et al., 2006; Bacon, 2002; Marcellin, Levy et al., 1997). Therefore, patients with chronic HCV and normal ALT levels should undergo further testing to determine indication for treatment.

A liver biopsy is recommended to assess the severity of inflammation and fibrosis, but is not mandatory before starting treatment. Since individuals with genotypes 2 and 3 have a high response rate, treatment may be initiated for these patients without a liver biopsy. However, it is essential to determine a patient's genotype and viral load before initiating treatment (Sherman et al., 2007). The HCV genotype determines the duration of treatment and affects the response rate.

Standard pharmacotherapy for HCV

Based on randomized controlled trials, a new regimen of once-weekly injection of pegylated interferon (PEG IFN) plus daily oral ribavirin has become the standard of care for the initial treatment of chronic HCV infection (Manns et al., 2001; Zaman et al., 2003; Hadziyannis et al., 2004; Sherman et al., 2007). This approach has a similar safety profile to the previously standard interferon-based combination therapy, but with a statistically better SVR (sustained virologic response), which is defined as the absence of HCV RNA in the serum six months after the end of treatment.

Patients with genotype 1 are usually treated for 48 weeks and have an SVR of 42 to 51 per cent (Jaeckel et al., 2001; Craxi & Licata, 2003; Hadziyannis et al., 2004). In comparison, patients with genotype 2 or 3 have a 78 to 82 per cent likelihood of responding after 24 weeks of therapy. Viral load also affects SVR, with better response rates being achieved with lower viral loads (Sherman et al., 2004; Fried, 2004). Patients who respond to treatment have a minimal chance (about two per cent) of relapse and tend to have a reduced rate of progression to cirrhosis and HCC (Almasio et al., 2003; Marcellin, Boyer et al., 1997).

Treatment response is monitored by measuring HCV RNA concentrations. An early virological response (EVR) can be used to predict the chance of an SVR in patients with genotype 1 infection (Fried, 2004; Davis et al., 2003). EVR is defined as an undetectable level of HCV RNA, or a greater than 2 log decrease from baseline concentration levels, at 12 weeks of treatment. Patients with genotype 1 who fail to demonstrate an EVR have less than a three per cent chance of achieving an SVR, so therapy should be discontinued in these cases. Patients who experience a greater than 2 log drop at 12 weeks should be assessed again with a qualitative HCV RNA at 24 weeks—if they have not cleared the virus at this point, therapy should be withdrawn since the patients are unlikely to achieve an SVR. Patients with genotype 2 or 3 have an EVR in 97 per cent of cases and do not need testing at 12 weeks of therapy.

Absolute contraindications to combined therapy include poor adherence, decompensated liver disease, ongoing substance abuse, pregnancy and certain co-existing medical conditions (such as uncontrolled seizure disorder, uncontrolled severe psychiatric disorder or certain autoimmune diseases, including autoimmune hepatitis and systemic lupus erythematosus) (Wong & Lee, 2006).

Patients undergoing combination therapy need close monitoring for complications and should undergo regular laboratory assessments (a recommended schedule of evaluations is presented in Table 14-1 on page 128). Table 14-2 outlines the common side-effects of the pegylated interferon and ribarivin regimen (all of which occur in more than 10 per cent of cases). Sexually active patients undergoing combination therapy should be advised to use an effective method of contraception for the duration of treatment and for six months following treatment completion (Sherman et al., 2007).

New regimens for treatment of hepatitis C

Recent recommendations focus on changing the duration of treatment based on results of rapid virological response (RVR) testing, which is defined as the absence of HCV RNA at week four (Sherman et al., 2007). RVR is thought to be the best predictor of SVR.

Therefore, using RVR, patients with genotype 1 infection who achieve RVR may be treated to 24 weeks. Treatment for 48 weeks is indicated if a relapse occurs. Treatment may be extended to 72 weeks for those with only a partial virological response (PVR).

TABLE 14-1

Monitoring during combination treatment

LABORATORY EVALUATION	FREQUENCY
CBC	at 1, 2, 4, 6, 8 weeks, then monthly
AST, ALT, ALP, bilirubin, INR, albumin, creatinine, TSH, glucose, urinalysis	every 3 months
Pregnancy test	periodically

Adapted with permission from Sherman et al., 2007. This material was originally published in *Canadian Journal of Gastroenterology* 2007:21 (Suppl C): 25C–34C.

TABLE 14-2

Common side-effects of HCV treatment regimen

INTERFERON	RIBAVIRIN
mild bone marrow suppression (anemia, leukopenia, thrombocytopenia)	hemolytic anemia (dose dependent)
insomnia, depression	fatigue
fatigue, irritability	rash and pruritus
weight loss, anorexia	nasal stuffiness
alopecia	cough
skin irritation at injection site	
nausea, vomiting, diarrhea	
fever, myalgia, flu-like symptoms, headaches	

Wong & Lee, 2006. © Canadian Medical Association. This work is protected by copyright and the making of this copy was with the permission of Access Copyright. Any alteration of its content or further copying in any form whatsoever is strictly prohibited unless otherwise permitted by law.

For patients with genotype 2 and 3 infections, RVR indicates a high chance of SVR at 12 to 16 weeks. Retreatment for 24 weeks is advised in the case of relapse.

Retreatment options

Previous antiviral therapies of standard interferon and ribavirin have been associated with more treatment failure due to a variety of factors. It is important to distinguish between patients who do not respond to treatment and those who do respond but relapse (Sherman et al., 2004). Relapsers show no HCV RNA during treatment, but experience a reappearance of the virus after the withdrawal of therapy. Non-responders do not eliminate HCV RNA with treatment. For both groups, retreatment with PEG IFN and ribavirin combination therapy should be offered (Sherman et al., 2007). Reports indicate that 20 per cent of relapsers and 10 per cent of non-responders are likely to achieve an SVR (Shiffman, 2002) if retreated.

SUMMARY

Physicians have a vital role to play in screening patients who are at high risk for hepatitis C, especially patients who use injection drugs. All HCV-positive patients should undergo evaluation for treatment and should be counselled about preventing further transmission. Avoiding hepatotoxic agents such as alcohol and receiving hepatitis A and B vaccinations can slow the progression of HCV to cirrhosis and HCC.

Overcoming the barriers and complications associated with HCV treatment can be challenging for some patients, especially among substance-using populations. Methadone-prescribing physicians need to work with other health care providers in supporting substance users' access to complete HCV treatment.

Other chronic medical conditions

A few other concurrent conditions are worth briefly mentioning here.

Hepatic disease

Case reports suggest that hepatic impairment does not cause an increase in serum methadone levels, and does not put patients at greater risk for hepatic toxicity. However, in our clinical experience, patients who develop acute hepatic deficiency or hepatorenal syndrome are at increased risk for methadone toxicity even if their dose is stable. As a precaution, patients with advanced liver disease should be titrated slowly on methadone. Benzodiazepines should be avoided in this population because their half-life may be prolonged in patients with hepatic dysfunction and because they can trigger hepatic encephalopathy.

Renal disease

The metabolism of methadone is not altered by renal disease. However, as mentioned above, patients in acute renal failure may be at risk for toxicity. Methadone is highly protein bound and is not removed by dialysis.

Respiratory disease

Methadone should be titrated slowly and carefully in patients with underlying lung disease, since tolerance to its respiratory-depressant effects develops slowly. Methadone withdrawal may exacerbate acute respiratory conditions by causing anxiety and agitation.

Cardiac disease

Methadone is safe in patients with cardiac disease, except that high doses have been associated with torsades de pointes. Rapid methadone withdrawal should be avoided in patients with coronary artery disease.

References

Addiction Treatment Forum. (2005). *Methadone drug interactions.* Available: www.atforum.com.

Alberti, A., Noventa, F., Benvegnù, L., Boccato, S. & Gatta, A. (2002). Prevalence of liver disease in a population of asymptomatic persons with hepatitis C virus infection. *Annals of Internal Medicine, 137* (12), 961–964.

Almasio, P.L., Venezia, G. & Craxi, A. (2003). The impact of antiviral therapy on the course of chronic HCV infection: A systematic review. *Panminerva Medica, 45* (3), 175–182.

Alter, M.J., Kuhnert, W.L. & Finelli, L. (2003). Guidelines for laboratory testing and result reporting of antibody to hepatitis C virus. Centers for Disease Control and Prevention. *MMWR Recommendations and Reports, 52* (RR-3), 1–13, 15, quiz CE1–4.

Anderson J.F. (2000). Interpreting the relation between injection drug use and harm: A cautionary note. *Canadian Medical Association Journal, 162* (12), 1695–1696.

Andonov, A. & Chaudhary, R.K. (1994). Genotyping of Canadian hepatitis C virus isolates by PCR. *Journal of Clinical Microbiology, 32* (8), 2031–2034.

Antela, A. (2001). Access to antiretroviral therapy in HIV-infected injection drug users. *AIDS, 15,* 1727–1728.

Bacon, B.R. (2002). Treatment of patients with hepatitis C and normal serum aminotransferase levels. *Hepatology, 36* (5, suppl. 1), s179–s184.

Canadian Liver Foundation. (2000). Hepatitis C: Medical information update. *Canadian Journal of Public Health, 91* (suppl. 1), s4–s9.

Canadian Paediatric Society. (2008). Vertical transmission of the hepatitis C virus: Current knowledge and issues. *Paediatrics and Child Health, 13* (6), 529–534.

Clarke S.M. & Mulcahy, F.M. (2003). What's new for injection drug users with HIV infection? *Sexually Transmitted Infections, 79,* 80–83.

Craxi, A. & Licata, A. (2003). Clinical trial results of peginterferons in combination with ribavirin. *Seminars in Liver Disease, 23* (suppl. 1), 35–46.

Davis, G.L., Wong, J.B., McHutchinson, J.G., Manns, M.P., Harvey, J. & Albrecht, J. (2003). Early virologic response to treatment with peginterferon alfa-2b plus ribavirin in patients with chronic hepatitis C. *Hepatology, 38* (3), 645–652.

Dybul, M., Fauci, A.S., Bartlett, J.G., Kaplan, J.E. & Pau, A.K. (2002). Guidelines for using antiretroviral agents in HIV-1 infected adults and adolescents. *Annals of Internal Medicine, 137* (5), 381–433.

Donaher, P.A. & Welsh, C. (2006). Managing opioid addiction with buprenorphine. *American Family Physician, 73,* 1573–1578.

Edlin, B.R., Kresina, T.F., Raymond, D.B., Carden, M.R., Gourevitch, M.N., Rich, J.D. et al. (2005). Overcoming barriers to prevention, care, and treatment of hepatitis C in illicit drug users. *Clinical Infectious Diseases, 40* (suppl. 5), s276–s285.

Fried, M.W. (2004). Viral factors affecting the outcome of therapy for chronic hepatitis C. *Reviews in Gastroenterological Disorders, 4* (suppl. 1), s8–s13.

Gerlach, J.T., Diepolder, H.M., Zachoval, R., Gruener, N.H., Jung, M.C., Ulsenheimer, A. et al. (2003). Acute hepatitis C: High rate of both spontaneous and treatment-induced viral clearance. *Gastroenterology, 125* (1), 80–88.

Gowing, L., Farrell, M., Bornemann, R., Sullivan, L. & Ali, R. (2004). Substitution treatment of injecting opioid users for prevention of HIV infection (review*). Cochrane Database of Systematic Reviews, 4.*

Hadziyannis, S.J., Sette, H. Jr., Morgan, T.R., Balan, V., Diago, M., Marcellin, P. et al. (2004). Peginterferon-alpha2a and ribavirin combination therapy in chronic hepatitis C: A randomized study of treatment duration and ribavirin dose. *Annals of Internal Medicine, 140* (5), 346–355.

Health Canada. (2001). *Reducing the Harm Associated with Injection Drug Use in Canada.* Ottawa: Author. Available: www.hc-sc.gc.ca/hc-ps/pubs/adp-apd/injection/index-eng.php.

Hino, K., Sainokami, S., Shimoda, K., Niwa, H. & Iino, S. (1994). Clinical course of acute hepatitis C and changes in HCV markers. *Digestive Diseases and Sciences, 39* (1), 19–27.

Hoofnagle, J.H. (1997). Hepatitis C: The clinical spectrum of disease. *Hepatology, 26* (3, suppl. 1), 15s–20s.

Jaeckel, E., Cornberg, M., Wedemeyer, H., Santantonio, T., Mayer, J., Zankel, M. et al., (2001). Treatment of acute hepatitis C with interferon alfa-2b. *New England Journal of Medicine, 345* (20), 1452–1457.

Jauncey, M., Micallef, J.M., Gilmour, S., Amin, J., White, P.A., Rawlinson, W. et al. (2004). Clearance of hepatitis C virus after newly acquired infection in injection drug users. *Journal of Infectious Diseases, 190,* 1270–1274.

Kamal, S.M., Moustafa, K.N., Chen, J., Fehr, J., Abdel Moneim, A., Khalifa, K.E. et al. (2006). Duration of peginterferon therapy in acute hepatitis C: A randomized trial. *Hepatology, 43,* 923–931.

Kerr T., Stoltz, J., Strathdee, S., Li, K., Hogg, R.S., Montaner, J.S. et al. (2006). The impact of sex partners' HIV status on HIV seroconversion in a prospective cohort of injection drug users. *Journal of Acquired Immune Deficiency Syndromes, 41*, 119–123.

Manns, M.P., McHutchison, J.G., Gordon, S.C., Rustgi, V.K., Shiffman, M., Reindollar, R. et al. (2001). Peginterferon alfa-2b plus ribavirin compared with interferon alfa-2b plus ribavirin for initial treatment of chronic hepatitis C: A randomised trial. *The Lancet, 358* (9286), 958–965.

Marcellin, P., Boyer, N., Gervais, A., Martinot, M., Pouteau, M., Castelnau, C. et al. (1997). Long-term histologic improvement and loss of detectable intrahepatic HCV RNA in patients with chronic hepatitis C and sustained response to interferon-alpha therapy. *Annals of Internal Medicine, 127* (10), 875–881.

Marcellin, P., Levy, S. & Erlinger, S. (1997). Therapy of hepatitis C: Patients with normal aminotransferase levels. *Hepatology, 26* (3, suppl. 1), s133–s136.

March, D.C. (2000). HIV and substance use. In B. Brands (Ed.), *Management of Alcohol, Tobacco and Other Drug Problems: A Physician's Manual.* Toronto: Centre for Addiction and Mental Health.

Mathurin, P., Moussalli, J., Cadranel, J.F., Thibault, V., Charlotte, F., Dumouchel, P. et al. (1998). Slow progression rate of fibrosis in hepatitis C virus patients with persistently normal alanine transaminase activity. *Hepatology, 27* (3), 868–872.

Mattick, R.P., Breen, C., Kimber, J. & Davoli, M. (2003). Methadone maintenance therapy versus no opioid replacement therapy for opioid dependence (review). *Cochrane Database of Systematic Reviews, 2.*

Millson, P., Myers, T., Calzavara, L., Wallace, E., Major, C. & Degani, N. (2003). Regional variation in HIV prevalence and risk behaviours in Ontario injection drug users (IDU). *Canadian Journal of Public Health, 94* (6), 431–435.

NIH Consensus Statement on Management of Hepatitis C. (2002). *NIH Consensus and State-of-the-Science Statements, 19* (3), 1–46.

Pawlotsky, J.M. (2002). Use and interpretation of virological tests for hepatitis C. *Hepatology 36* (5, suppl. 1), s65–s73.

Public Health Agency of Canada. (2005). *HIV and AIDS in Canada: Surveillance Report to June 30, 2005.* Ottawa. Available: www.phac-aspc.gc.ca/publicat/aids-sida/haic-vsac0605/index-eng.php.

Research Group on Drug Use. (2004). *Drug Use in Toronto* (13th ed.). Available: www.toronto.ca/health/rgdu/index.htm. Retrieved August 2007.

Seeff, L.B. (1997). Natural history of hepatitis C. *Hepatology, 26* (3, suppl. 1), s21–s28.

Sherman, M., Bain, V., Villeneuve, J.P., Myers, R.P., Cooper, C., Martin, S. et al., (2004). The management of chronic viral hepatitis: A Canadian consensus conference. *Canadian Journal of Gastroenterology, 18* (12), 715–728.

Sherman, M., Shafran, S., Burak, K., Doucette, K., Wong, W., Gigrah, N. et al. (2007). Management of chronic hepatitis C: Consensus guidelines. *Canadian Journal of Gastroenterology, 21* (suppl. C), 25C–34C.

Shiffman, M.L. (2002). Retreatment of patients with chronic hepatitis C. *Hepatology, 36* (5, suppl. 1), s128–s134.

Shiffman, M.L., Diago, M., Tran, A., Pockros, P., Reindollar, R., Prati, D. et al. (2006). Chronic hepatitis C in patients with persistently normal alanine transaminase levels. *Clinical Gastroenterology and Hepatology, 4*, 645–652.

Strathdee, S.A., Patrick, D.M., Currie, S.L., Cornelisse, P.G., Rekart, M.L., Montaner, J.S. et al. (1997). Needle exchange is not enough: Lessons from the Vancouver injecting drug use study. *AIDS, 11*, f59–f65.

Tessier, D., Dion, H., Grossman, D.W. & Rachlis, A. (2001). *HIV Care: A Primer and Resource for Family Physicians.* Mississauga, ON: College of Family Physicians of Canada.

Tyndall, M.W., Patrick, D., Spittal, P., Lik, K., O'Shaughnessy, M. & Schechter, M. (2002). Risky sexual behaviours among injection drugs users with high HIV prevalence: Implications for STD control. *Sexually Transmitted Infections, 78* (suppl. i), i170–i175.

Wiegand, J., Buggisch, P., Boecher, W., Zeuzem, S., Gelbmann, C., Berg, T. et al. (2006). Early monotherapy with pegylated interferon alpha-2b for acute hepatitis C infection: The HEP-NET acute-HCV-II study. *Hepatology, 43*, 250–256.

Wong, T. & Lee, S.S. (2006). Hepatitis C: A review for primary care physicians. *Canadian Medical Association Journal, 174* (5), 649–659.

Wood, E., Tyndall, M.W., Spittal, P.M., Li, K., Kerr, T., Hogg, R.S. et al. (2001). Unsafe injection practices in a cohort of injection drug users in Vancouver: Could safer injecting rooms help? *Canadian Medical Association Journal, 165* (4), 405–410.

Wood, E., Hogg, R.S., Kerr, T., Palepu, A., Zhang, R. & Montaner, J.S. (2005). Impact of accessing methadone on the time to initiating HIV treatment among antiretroviral-naive HIV-infected injection drug users. *AIDS, 19* (8), 837–839.

Yeni, P.G., Hammer, S.M., Hirsch, M.S., Saag, M.S., Schechter, M. & Carpenter, C.C. (2004). Treatment for adult HIV-infection: 2004 recommendations of the international AIDS society—USA panel. *Journal of the American Medical Association, 292* (2), 251–265.

Zaman, A., Fennerty, M.B. & Keeffe, E.B. (2003). Systematic review: Peginterferon vs. standard interferon in the treatment of chronic hepatitis C. *Alimentary Pharmacology and Therapeutics. 18* (7): 661–670.

Zarski, J.P. & Leroy, V. (1999). Counselling patients with hepatitis C. *Journal of Hepatology, 31* (suppl. 1), 136–140.

Zou, S., Tepper, M. & Giulivi, A. (2000). Current status of hepatitis C in Canada. *Canadian Journal of Public Health, 91* (suppl. 1), s10–5, S10–6.

CHAPTER 15

Pregnancy and opioid use

This chapter outlines the specific needs and considerations of women who are using opioids and become pregnant. It begins with general information about pregnancy and opioid use, and explains the relevant medical assessment and management. It also discusses the special needs and challenges of women who use substances and their difficulty accessing care. Finally, the chapter describes how to initiate and maintain MMT in pregnant patients and how to manage neonatal abstinence syndrome.

Background

Opioid use during pregnancy is considered a high-risk condition in terms of perinatal management, and pregnant women in MMT need to be monitored attentively.

Most women using heroin and other opioids are of childbearing age, although the exact incidence of pregnancy in this population is unknown, as is the incidence of pregnancy in MMT-maintained women. Any physician who prescribes methadone may at some time receive a request to assess a pregnant woman who uses opioids.

Managing a pregnancy together with opioid dependence can begin with any one of the following three situations:

- a pregnant woman who is not yet being treated for her opioid use presents for MMT
- a woman stabilized on methadone becomes pregnant
- a pregnant woman presents with a past history of opioid dependence, although she is not using now.

Approximately one per cent of women of childbearing age use opioids. Because of the amenorrhea associated with use, many of these women believe that their opioid dependence confers protection against pregnancy. While the amenorrhea is secondary to anovulation (Reisine & Pasternack, 1996), some women who use opioids do ovulate, especially when there is a reduction in opioid use. It is important to rule out an undiagnosed pregnancy as a cause of secondary amenorrhea in women who use opioids at the first presentation for treatment.

Women who are being stabilized on methadone may become pregnant (Finnegan, 1979). This is because the FSH-LH axis begins to function normally, leading to the return of ovulation (Santen et al., 1975). Some form of birth control should therefore be recommended for women entering MMT in order to prevent an unwanted pregnancy. If a woman on stable doses of methadone misses a menstrual period, she should have a pregnancy test.

Effects of opioid use during pregnancy

EFFECTS ON THE FETUS

Evidence suggests that heroin is not a human teratogen and that there is no significant difference in the frequency of congenital anomalies in children of women who have used heroin during pregnancy (Little et al., 1990). Nevertheless, pregnant women who are opioid dependent have high infant morbidity and mortality rates, primarily because of the high rates of prematurity and low birth weight (Rementeria & Nunag 1973; Finnegan, 1978; Kandall et al., 1977; Wilson et al., 1981; Stimmel et al., 1983; Little et al., 1990; Hulse et al., 1997; Hulse et al., 1998).

Low birth weight has been attributed to the direct effects of heroin on the fetus. Other factors that contribute to low birth weight include poor nutrition, smoking and inadequate prenatal care (Hulse et al., 1997).

EFFECTS ON THE MOTHER

Women who are pregnant and using heroin may be more likely to experience medical complications during their pregnancies than other women because of factors such as the method of drug use (i.e., injection), opioid withdrawal and lack of prenatal care. A variety of infections are highly prevalent in this population, including hepatitis, urinary tract infections, cellulitis, sexually transmitted infections, septicemia and bacterial endocarditis (Stern, 1966; Finnegan, 1991; Vucinovic et al., 2008).

Obstetrical complications, associated with opioid withdrawal and lack of prenatal care, are also more frequent in women who are opioid dependent (Finnegan, 1991; Hulse et al., 1998). Opioid withdrawal can trigger uterine contractions, which may lead to spontaneous abortion in the first trimester and premature labour in the third trimester (Finnegan, 1991). The effects of opioid use in pregnancy are complicated by the variety of personal and family problems that are encountered by this population. Women who are opioid dependent often have a history of mental health issues, including physical and sexual abuse and mood disorders (Currie, 2001). Low levels of education along with inadequate housing and financial resources can compound these challenges (Kaltenbach et al., 1998).

Rationale for MMT during pregnancy

Methadone is the treatment of choice for opioid dependence in pregnancy. MMT should be offered to all pregnant women who are dependent on opioids. Its advantages include the following:

- better prenatal care
- better nutrition
- reduced opioid withdrawal and cravings
- reduced use of other illicit substances
- reduced incidence of preterm delivery
- increased birth weight
- decreased infant mortality (Kaltenbach & Finnegan, 1992; Chang et al. 1992).

Regular prenatal care, counselling, prenatal classes designed for this population, and co-ordination of services such as child care and parenting classes are necessary adjuncts to the provision of methadone to pregnant patients. A higher number of prenatal visits and enhanced treatment for opioid-dependent women are associated with improved neonatal outcomes (Chang et al., 1992).

Effects of methadone on the fetus and infant

Methadone crosses the placenta but is not considered to be a teratogen (Blinick et al., 1974). However, evidence suggests that there is an increased occurrence of strabismus in infants born to opioid-dependent women, especially in those exposed antenatally to methadone (Nelson et al., 1987; Gill et al., 2003).

Among infants born to methadone-maintained mothers there is a high incidence of neonatal abstinence syndrome (NAS) (Kaltenbach & Finnegan, 1986).

Studies have demonstrated variable findings related to the association between intrauterine growth restriction and methadone treatment. Some studies have found that infants born to mothers in MMT tend to have smaller head circumferences, length and lower birth weights (Wilson et al., 1981; Chasnoff et al., 1982; Lifschitz et al., 1985; Kaltenbach & Finnegan, 1987; Edelin et al., 1988; Hans, 1989), but these differences disappeared within a year or two of follow-up (Vance et al., 1997; Lifschitz et al., 1985; Hunt et al., 2008). However, studies have reported that infants born to women in MMT had higher birth weights than those born to women who were using heroin throughout pregnancy (Zelson et al., 1973; Kandall et al., 1976; Connaughton et al., 1977; Lifschitz et al., 1985; Giles et al., 1989).

The effects of antenatal exposure to opioids, specifically methadone, on long-term development remain uncertain (Chasnoff et al., 1982; Lifschitz et al., 1985; Kaltenbach & Finnegan, 1987; Hans, 1989). The literature suggests that infants exposed to opioids in utero may be at increased risk for poorer neurodevelopmental outcomes (e.g., motor and/or cognitive delays) (Hans, 1989; Hunt et al., 2008). However, environmental factors and caregivers play a significant role in mediating growth and developmental outcomes for these infants.

Diagnosis and treatment

PRESENTING FOR CARE

Many women who become pregnant while using opioids first present for an initial obstetrics consultation in the second or third trimester after having discovered their pregnant condition around the time of quickening or when abdominal distension was becoming evident. Some opioid-dependent women may only present for care when in labour. A diagnosis of opioid use during labour should be suspected when the woman's presentation suggests physical withdrawal or intoxication, or the woman requires and tolerates unusually large doses of opioid analgesia. Less often, the diagnosis of a pregnant woman's opioid dependence is only made in the postpartum period when the neonate develops withdrawal symptoms.

INDICATORS OF OPIOID DEPENDENCE

The obstetrical care provider should suspect substance use if one or more of the following behaviours are observed:

- frequent failures to attend antenatal appointments
- requests for opioids
- complications typical of injection drug use
- signs of intoxication or withdrawal
- unexplained poor obstetric outcomes in the past, including stillbirth
- indications of intrauterine growth restriction
- signs of premature labour.

A woman may disclose opioid use to her obstetrical care provider if she is asked directly about substance use in a non-judgmental manner.

GUIDELINES FOR ASSESSMENT

Pregnant women who are opioid dependent often have multiple medical problems and unique psychosocial needs, in addition to being at high risk for maternal and neonatal complications. A comprehensive assessment of the substance use, associated consequences and circumstances of a pregnant woman who has opioid dependence should include the following areas.

Substance use history

The patient's substance use history, including any current symptoms of withdrawal, needs to be determined. The physician should inquire about the use of prescription and over-the-counter opioid analgesics and sedatives in addition to cannabis, tobacco and alcohol.

Taking the drug history will also help the clinician assess the degree and type of physical and psychosocial complications, which will help in the formulation of a treatment plan. The woman should be asked directly about risk factors for hepatitis C transmission, including injection drug use and sharing drug paraphernalia.

Obstetric history

The outcomes of previous pregnancies are a rich source of information in designing the treatment plan with the patient.

Psychiatric history

The patient needs to be screened for depression, anxiety and eating disorders, and any appropriate treatment should be offered.

History of sexual, physical, and/or emotional abuse

Prior and current sexual, physical and/or emotional abuse is very common. Physicians should elicit this history specifically, since pregnancy is an especially high-risk time for experiencing flashbacks of previous abuse and for the initiation of abuse by partners.

Psychosocial assessment

A comprehensive psychosocial assessment should be conducted, paying attention to areas of special relevance to pregnancy. The physician should determine the woman's current living arrangements, partner and vocational status. The patient's partner may also require treatment for substance use.

A nutritional assessment should also be included. It is important to inquire into the woman's source of food, since some women rely on local food banks.

Also ask pregnant women about parenting

arrangements and the safety of children living at home. It is important to enquire about any involvement of child protective services with her other children.

It is useful to have a list of local social service agencies to which the woman can be referred, if appropriate.

Medical history

In taking the medical history, it is very important to ask about any history of hepatitis B and C and/or HIV infection.

RECOMMENDED MEDICAL TESTS

Urine drug screens

A urine drug screen should be done to confirm the diagnosis of opioid dependence. Obtain informed consent prior to ordering any urine drug screen testing.

A woman who is opioid dependent should have at least twice-weekly urine drug screens for the first eight weeks to test for drugs of abuse prevalent in the local community.

Patients who become stable can have random urine drug screens every one to two weeks. During pregnancy, urine drug screens should be observed. Alternatively, routine temperature testing or urine pH and creatinine levels can be measured to assess for sample tampering.

Test for infections

Particular attention should be paid to the Pap smear and cervico-vaginal cultures. Indications for tuberculosis and viral hepatitis screening should also be considered. Pregnant women with high-risk behaviours should be retested for sexually transmitted infections throughout the pregnancy.

HIV-positive patients

Discussing and offering HIV testing to all pregnant women has become the standard of care. Prompt diagnosis of HIV is recommended to allow the introduction of chemoprophylaxis, which has been shown to reduce vertical transmission to the fetus. With treatment, the chance of vertical transmission is reduced from 25 per cent to approximately eight per cent (Connor et al., 1994). Early diagnosis and treatment can also improve maternal outcomes (Connor et al., 1994). Women who continue with injection drug use and high-risk sexual practices during the pregnancy should be offered testing repeatedly, especially in the third trimester.

Prenatal testing

All routine gestation-specific tests should be ordered. An ultrasound is usually indicated to estimate gestational age, since most women who are opioid dependent are not aware of the first day of their last menstrual cycle.

Third-trimester surveillance

Methadone-maintained pregnancies may need more frequent clinical visits to monitor for signs of premature labour and to assess fetal growth. Repeated ultrasound testing may be indicated for growth measurements. Additional antenatal fetal surveillance may be initiated based on past obstetrical history and current maternal or fetal conditions requiring monitoring instead of substance use history alone. In addition, these risk factors will determine the method and frequency of testing (Liston et al., 2007).

Continued heroin use in pregnancy has been associated with increased perinatal morbidity and mortality, especially increased risk of stillbirth and neonatal deaths secondary to prematurity (Fricker & Segal, 1978; Hulse et al., 1998; Fajemirokun-Odudeyi et al., 2006; Vucinovic et al., 2008). Therefore, antenatal surveillance may be indicated in these clinical situations.

Fetal surveillance in stable methadone-maintained women may only be indicated in the presence of risk factors such as intrauterine growth restriction. Exposure to methadone affects fetal performance on the non-stress test (NST) and the biophysical profile (BPP). These changes may limit the reliability of these tests in monitoring for fetal well-being in women who are pregnant and in MMT, especially if the methadone dosing interval is not taken into consideration when interpreting the test results.

NST (non-stress test)

Archie et al. (1989) first documented that methadone altered the morphology of the NST when the test is performed one hour after methadone ingestion. The reactivity was significantly decreased as shown by decreases in the frequencies of fetal movements and fetal heart rate accelerations.

These findings were supported by other studies demonstrating a higher incidence of non-reactive NSTS and a longer interval to achieve a reactive test in women who are pregnant and in MMT (Levine & Rebarber, 1995; Anyaegbunam et al., 1997). These changes have been linked to methadone effects despite the concomitant use of nicotine and other substances.

The optimal time for performing an NST relative to methadone dosing has yet to be determined.

BPP (biophysical profile)

Methadone has also been found to affect the BPP (Cejtin et al., 1996). Although the overall score was not significantly affected, the time needed to complete the BPP was longer after methadone dosing. Fetal breathing movement was the most commonly affected variable. It has been hypothesized that this outcome is related to a methadone-induced sleep state.

Initiating methadone

The guiding principle when discussing methadone with a pregnant woman who has been determined to be opioid dependent is to take a woman-centred approach rather than simply focusing on the pregnancy. Care providers should maintain a gentle, non-confrontational attitude when reviewing the benefits and risks of a pregnant woman's continued opioid use in comparison to methadone maintenance treatment. It is also important at this time to orient the patient to the rules of the MMT program. The physician should aim for the effective dose of methadone that is required to keep the patient comfortable for 24 hours and to maintain abstinence from other opioids. An appropriate maintenance dose needs to be found for each individual woman. A pregnant patient who has not previously been on methadone should be offered admission to the hospital where she can be monitored for withdrawal and fetal distress while her methadone dose is stabilized (Kaltenbach et al., 1998).

PROTOCOL FOR INPATIENT INITIATION

At the first sign of withdrawal, 10 to 20 mg of methadone is given as an initial dose, followed by additional 5 mg doses every four to six hours if withdrawal symptoms are present. On day two, the previous day's total dose is given as a single morning dose, followed by supplemental doses of 5 mg if withdrawal symptoms persist. Most patients can achieve symptom control on a daily dose of 20 to 35 mg after the first 48 to 72 hours (Finnegan 1991; Kaltenbach et al., 1998).

The dose is considered stable if no prn medications are required over a 24-hour period. Most patients are discharged on doses of 35 to 60 mg. Stabilization on methadone usually requires five to seven days.

The need for subsequent dosage increases as an outpatient should be carefully assessed, and increments should be no more than 5 to 10 mg. However, patients who continue to experience significant withdrawal symptoms or who continue to use other opioids should be offered an increased dose of methadone. The known risks of continued illicit opioid use outweigh the potential risks of higher doses of methadone. Subsequently, many patients may need a 10–30 mg increase in their methadone dose during the pregnancy (Finnegan, 1991). During the initial hospital stay, investigations necessary to evaluate the patient's health and prenatal status should be performed. The patient should also meet the rest of the team that will be managing both her pregnancy and her opioid dependence, including the following care providers: social worker, counsellor, obstetrical care provider, neonatologist or physician providing care for the methadone-exposed infant, and nursery and labour-room staff.

PROTOCOL FOR OUTPATIENT INITIATION

Often stabilization is accomplished on an outpatient basis because admission to hospital is not feasible. Several patient factors can make admission impractical, including:

- a patient's fear of medical personnel or hospitals
- child-care issues
- lack of supportive partner
- systemic factors, such as lack of services, non-availability of methadone in the hospital and hospital staff's limited experience in treating this population.

No formal studies exist to demonstrate the efficacy and safety of inpatient over outpatient stabilization. Outpatient initiation should only be undertaken after a discussion of the potential risks and benefits.

The following outpatient protocol was devised by Hoegerman and Schnoll (1991). It requires frequent reassessment of the patient and daily attendance at the clinic for dose adjustments. The patient is advised to arrive at the clinic for the first appointment of the morning. She is assessed for withdrawal and a urine drug screen sample is collected. A breathalyser test for alcohol is done, if necessary.

If withdrawal is mild or moderate, a starting dose of 15 mg of methadone is administered orally. The patient is observed for several hours for intoxication. The patient then returns in the late afternoon and is reassessed for intoxication or withdrawal and medicated again with an additional dose of 5 to 10 mg of methadone. Permitting the patient to return after hours to the clinic or hospital if she experiences withdrawal may prevent use of other opioids.

On day two, the woman can receive the previous day's total dose as a single dose in the morning and, if she is still experiencing withdrawal, her total daily dose can be increased by 10 mg. It may still be necessary to offer prn medication for later on in the day. For subsequent days, the morning dose can be calculated by giving the previous day's 24-hour total dose as a single dose or by increasing the previous day's total dose by 10 mg. Caution should be exercised to prevent an overdose of methadone. A maximum dose of 35 mg of methadone by day three should not be exceeded. When initiating methadone on an outpatient basis, it may take weeks before a stable dose is reached. Once stable, the patient should be converted to once-daily dosing.

Alternatively, pregnant women who decline to return for monitoring on a daily basis can be initiated following the outpatient protocol for non-pregnant individuals. The initial dose can be 10 to 20 mg of methadone per day for the first three days. The dose can then be increased by 5 to 15 mg every three to five days. The patient should be seen every three days to reassess response to the methadone dose and ongoing opioid use until a more stable dose of methadone is reached. If the pregnant woman complains of uterine irritability, including abdominal cramping and bleeding, then admission to hospital is indicated to monitor for signs of threatened spontaneous abortion or preterm labour. This will also permit for a faster increase in her methadone dose while under close observation.

MAINTENANCE PHASE

Maintaining a pregnant woman on methadone on an outpatient basis should continue as with any other patient in MMT. The patient should be assessed every one to two weeks regarding her methadone dose—sooner if the clinical situation warrants. Missed doses should be replaced as for non-pregnant individuals.

Vomited doses should be replaced after appropriate evaluation by the prescribing physician according to the time between the dosing and emesis (see Table 15-1). The patient should be observed when taking the replacement dose. Repeated requests for replacement doses require assessment of the following: substance use, carry status and presence of medical conditions contributing to emesis. During pregnancy, adequate treatment of nausea and vomiting will decrease the frequency of vomited doses.

TABLE 15-1

Schedule for replacement doses post-emesis

TIME INTERVAL BETWEEN METHADONE DOSING AND EMESIS	ACTION
<15 minutes	Replace full dose
15–30 minutes	Replace 50% of dose
>30 minutes	Do not replace dose

Note: Pregnant women should not be allowed to experience opioid withdrawal due to potential risks.

Dose adjustments during pregnancy

Women in MMT prior to conception should remain on their pre-pregnancy doses during the first and second trimesters (Finnegan, 1991). Small dose increases are sometimes necessary in the third trimester. The clearance rate of methadone appears to gradually increase from the first to the third trimester, resulting in lower mean serum methadone levels as the pregnancy progresses (Jarvis et al., 1999; Drozdick et al., 2002; Wolff et al., 2005). Possible explanations for this altered methadone clearance are increased methadone metabolism during pregnancy, increased maternal renal elimination, increased volume of distribution and tissue binding and metabolism by placenta and fetus (Pond et al., 1985; Swift et al., 1989). Based on these studies, increasing the dose of methadone later in pregnancy will be necessary to prevent maternal withdrawal symptoms.

Dose splitting

An alternative to increasing the dose in the third trimester is to administer methadone in divided doses. Twice-daily methadone dosing has been associated with sustained plasma methadone levels and thus with fewer withdrawal symptoms (Swift et al., 1989; Wittmann & Segal, 1991). This effect also leads to increased treatment compliance and decreased use of other illicit drugs (Swift et al., 1989; DePetrillo & Rice, 1995). Dose splitting has also been shown to cause less suppression of fetal behaviour than single dosing, which has demonstrated significant decreases in both body movements and breathing after dosing (Wittmann & Segal, 1991; Jansson et al., 2009). When single dose treatment continues to produce maternal withdrawal symptoms, twice-daily dosing (i.e., every 12 hours) can be considered.

This strategy is ideal for women who are stable for take-home dosing. If there are any concerns about the patient taking home the evening dose of methadone, arrangements should be made for a local pharmacy to dispense the evening dose as an observed dose.

DISCONTINUING METHADONE DURING PREGNANCY

Discontinuing methadone during pregnancy should be avoided if possible; however, maternal request to taper in order to eliminate the risk of neonatal withdrawal has to be considered. If tapering is attempted during the pregnancy, the safest time is between 14 and 32 weeks, when the risk of spontaneous abortion, premature labour and withdrawal-induced fetal stress is lowest (Finnegan, 1991; Kaltenbach et al., 1998). This recommendation is based on older data which showed that lowering the maternal methadone dose during the third trimester caused hyperactivity of both the fetal adrenal gland and the sympathetic nervous system secondary to intrauterine fetal withdrawal (Zuspan et al., 1975). Also, intrauterine fetal deaths were reported due to withdrawal from methadone in the late second trimester and last trimester (Zuspan et al., 1975; Rementeria & Nunag, 1973). Therefore, discontinuation of methadone during the third trimester was not advised. More recent clinical experience has failed to show an increased incidence of obstetrical complications or adverse neonatal outcomes with withdrawal from methadone during the first, second or third trimester (Blinick et al.,1969; Maas et al., 1990; Dashe et al., 1998; Luty et al., 2003; Jones et al., 2008).

However, clinical experience has shown that decreasing a patient's methadone dose can lead to instability and relapse; therefore, the decision to reduce a patient's dose should be made with care based on the patient's individual situation. Women who remained in MMT were more likely to remain in treatment longer and attend more obstetrical visits (Jones et al., 2008).

There is limited guidance in the literature on the process for medical withdrawal. Recommendations include reducing the dose by 1 to 2 mg per day as an inpatient or by 2 to 10 mg every one to two weeks as an outpatient (Finnegan 1991; Jarvis & Schnoll 1994; Archie 1998; Kandall et al., 1999).

These numbers are not based on systematic studies. In pregnancy, the dose should be decreased slowly; consider following the CPSO recommendations to reduce the dose by no more than five to 10 per cent per week (CPSO, 2005).

Managed withdrawal from methadone may be considered based on current obstetrical complications, duration and severity of opioid dependence and past treatment failures. Patients who have a short addiction history, medical stability, social stability with a good support network, and no concurrent psychiatric disorders may have better outcomes following discontinuation of methadone. The tapering should be stopped if any adverse consequences are reported, such as relapse to drug use or increased cravings or withdrawal symptoms, and if necessary, the methadone dose should be increased. Support and relapse prevention strategies should be employed with this population, since managed withdrawal is less effective than methadone maintenance treatment.

INTRAPARTUM MANAGEMENT

When a woman in MMT goes into labour, urine drug screening should be carried out with her consent as part of the routine admission assessment. It is important to review her viral hepatitis and HIV status and to include in the examination a search for active herpetic lesions.

The patient should be given her methadone dose for the day. If the woman needs to be on restricted oral intake for any reason, it should be dispensed in a reduced volume of fluid. Parenteral methadone is not available in Canada.

Neonatology or pediatrics staff should be informed about the impending birth. If the circumstances indicate, the appropriate child protective agency should be alerted.

Pain management

Methadone will not provide pain relief during the intrapartum period, so additional obstetric analgesia may be necessary. Methadone-maintained women are more likely to have increased pain sensitivity and higher reported pain scores due to chronic opioid administration (Scimeca et al., 2000; Mehta & Langford, 2006). The preferred method is epidural analgesia, but doses of pure opioid agonists, such as morphine, may be given if necessary. Current knowledge indicates that opioids are an effective and safe pain management option for pregnant women being treated for opioid dependence (Wunsch et al., 2003; Alford et al., 2006). Because of their tolerance to opioids, such women may require larger doses of the drug than most to achieve analgesia.

The only contraindicated opioids are mixed agonist/antagonists like pentazocine, which will precipitate acute withdrawal.

Fetal monitoring

Intermittent external electronic fetal monitoring is usually adequate. Any decision regarding the use of a fetal scalp clip for monitoring should be made after careful consideration of the risk of transmitting blood-borne diseases to the infant. As with any other delivery, universal body precautions should be maintained.

POSTPARTUM MANAGEMENT

In the early postpartum period, the mother should be offered analgesia over and above her baseline dose of methadone. Careful monitoring for postpartum depression is important. The mother often feels extremely guilty if the infant exhibits symptoms of withdrawal. Every effort should be made to encourage the mother to participate in the care of her child.

A few days or weeks postpartum, the mother may find her established dose of methadone to be too high. If so, it should be titrated down by 5 to 10 mg every week based on clinical symptoms until a new stable dose is reached. The minimum recommended postpartum duration for MMT is six months; the clinician should consider the danger to the mother and infant that could result from relapse to illicit opioids before beginning a taper.

The services of a visiting public health nurse are invaluable for patients in this population. Parenting classes should be offered to the mothers and their partners. Attendance at local drop-in centres should also be encouraged, as well as regular pediatric follow-up appointments.

Breastfeeding

Despite the barriers to breastfeeding faced by women in MMT, there are numerous benefits, such as promoting bonding between the mother and her infant and providing passive immunity to infection. Methadone enters the breast milk in very small amounts that are unlikely to be clinically significant (Jansson et al., 2004). The calculated mean daily methadone ingested by infants ranges between 0.01 and 0.05 mg depending on maternal methadone dose. This amount is not sufficient to prevent NAS and the infant may still require additional opioid treatment for withdrawal symptoms and signs. Therefore, breastfeeding during methadone maintenance is considered safe regardless of maternal dose (Jansson et al., 2004; Glatstein et al., 2008).

Women who are using other drugs in the postpartum period should be counselled regarding the risks of drug exposure to infants. Additional information is available from Motherisk (416 813-6780) or other clinical resources (Briggs et al., 2005).

In North America, the only absolute contraindication to breastfeeding is HIV. Breastfeeding by women who have acquired hepatitis C (HCV) is considered safe, as no studies have demonstrated the transmission of HCV through breast milk alone (Wong & Lee, 2006).

REPORTING TO CHILD PROTECTION AGENCIES

In Ontario, the *Child and Family Services Act* is intended to promote the best interests, protection and well-being of children. Any health care professional who has reasonable grounds to suspect that a child is, or may be, in need of protection has a legal duty to report this suspicion. The decision to make a referral to the appropriate child protection agency depends on the length of time the mother has been in treatment, the stability of her methadone dose and her social stability. Patients should be encouraged to self-report during the prenatal period.

If the child protection agency staff have appropriate training concerning MMT, they are unlikely to automatically apprehend a child whose mother is an MMT patient. If the child's home environment is stable and the mother has stopped using illicit drugs, the agency will generally instead provide supervision and other services in the home.

Unfortunately, some pregnant women in MMT are not able to stabilize their lives prior to delivery, and in such cases the child protection agency may apprehend the child. If this occurs, it is a time of high risk for the mother for a complete relapse to drug use. Therefore, she will need a great deal of support and assistance to help her meet the requirements of the child protection agency for the safe return of her child.

Care of the methadone-exposed infant

NEONATAL ABSTINENCE SYNDROME (NAS)[1]

Methadone readily crosses the placenta. Up to 85 per cent of newborns exposed to methadone experience neonatal abstinence syndrome (NAS) (Finnegan et al., 1975), characterized by withdrawal symptoms and signs (Bell & Lau, 1995) of CNS hyperirritability (high-pitched cry, increased muscle tone, sleep disturbances, tremors, seizures), gastrointestinal dysfunction (poor feeding, vomiting), respiratory distress and autonomic symptoms (sneezing, yawning, fever). The withdrawal usually begins within 72 hours of birth, but late presentations (two to four weeks after birth) have been reported. Symptoms may last for several weeks or months. Preterm infants had some notable differences in terms of NAS (Doberczak, 1991). Symptoms presented one to two days later and were less severe than with in-term infants and thus were less likely to require pharmacotherapy. These differences may be attributed to the immaturity of the preterm CNS which prevents the clinical presentation of NAS.

A clear relationship between maternal methadone dose and the severity of NAS has not been established (Berghella et al., 2003; Kaltenbach & Comfort, 1997; Dashe et al., 2002; Doberczak et al., 1993). Studies have found conflicting results regarding an association between methadone dose and NAS. Infants experiencing NAS are at high risk for sepsis, hypoglycemia and intracerebral hemorrhage; all of these conditions can mimic signs of withdrawal, so it is recommended that they be ruled out before any signs are attributed to withdrawal.

It is important to consider the effect of other concomitant drug use on the presentation of neonatal withdrawal. Neonates born to mothers in MMT who also use benzodiazepines showed more severe neonatal withdrawal and required a longer duration of treatment (Berghella et al., 2003).

To date, no conclusive long-term study has been published about the long-term effects of neonatal exposure to methadone.

1 Much of this section is based on Kaltenbach & Finnegan, 1986, 1992 and Finnegan, 1983.

Managing NAS

All infants born to women on methadone should be observed for a minimum of four to five days under the care of a physician experienced in the assessment and treatment of withdrawal. It has been demonstrated that 96 per cent of those infants needing treatment for NAS were identified by four days of age. Untreated withdrawal in infants can lead to seizures, excessive weight loss, dehydration and even death.

A neonatal urine sample should be sent for a drug screen with parental consent shortly after birth. The baby should be monitored for signs of withdrawal using a NAS scale (discussed below and in Table 15-2). While morphine is the treatment of choice, phenobarbital may also be used to treat withdrawal symptoms. Based on the literature, up to approximately 50 per cent of infants may require pharmacotherapy for NAS (McCarthy et al., 2005). The following management recommendations are based on the Finnegan NAS scoring system. Other similar scoring tools are also available.

NAS SCALE

The Finnegan NAS scale, presented in Table 15-2 on page 143, is a 21-item scale designed to assess the severity of withdrawal symptoms and to titrate the dose of oral morphine according to the severity of neonatal withdrawal symptoms (Finnegan, 1975; Finnegan & Kaltenbach, 1992).

Caregiving physicians should initiate scoring within two hours of an infant's birth, and should continue scoring every two to four hours for four to five days, or as long as morphine treatment and weaning are necessary. Neonates should not be wakened to obtain an NAS score. An item is scored if it occurs at any time within a four-hour interval. Each symptom has been assigned a severity score and the total score is the sum of all symptoms observed during the scoring interval.

Nurses and pediatricians should receive some training in the use of the NAS scale. If marked discrepancies in scoring are noted among different caregivers, they should reach a consensus on the most appropriate score. If the hospital rarely treats neonatal withdrawal, the physician should consider referring the infant to a centre with more experience and consult with a physician familiar with withdrawal management.

INITIATION OF MORPHINE

Morphine is administered as a scheduled fixed dose. The initial dose is determined by the infant's body weight and NAS score. Morphine administration is not meant to be determined on a sliding scale (like hyperglycemia and regular insulin), nor is it meant to be given on an as-needed basis. Morphine is not indicated if consecutive NAS scores, or the average of any three consecutive scores, is 7 or less. An average score of 8 or greater for three consecutive readings indicates the need for oral morphine.

Weaning from morphine

The neonate should continue on the dose of morphine that keeps the scores at 8 or less for 24 to 48 hours before weaning commences (Finnegan, 1975).

These guidelines should be followed when weaning an infant from morphine in the context of NAS:

- Weaning should continue as long as scores remain below 8.
- Weaning is usually by 0.05 mg/kg of daily dose, every two to four days (Finnegan, 1975).
- Morphine can be discontinued when the neonate is stable for two to four days on a dose as low as 0.05 to 0.1 mg/kg per day.
- Duration of weaning is usually two to eight weeks.

DISCHARGE FROM HOSPITAL

All neonates whose mothers have taken methadone in pregnancy should stay in hospital for at least four to five days and be discharged only if they show no signs of withdrawal or score lower than 8 on the NAS scale. If morphine treatment is initiated, the infant must remain in hospital until fully weaned off morphine and no longer in withdrawal.

At the time of discharge, mothers should be carefully instructed to watch for signs of withdrawal and to call immediately if they occur. The infant should be assessed again within one to two days of discharge.

It is extremely important to monitor the infant for delayed withdrawal. The infant can be extremely fussy or jittery, or have a hyperactive Moro reflex for an extended period of time. If the infant is feeding and gaining weight appropriately, simple conservative management is required. If not, the infant should be readmitted to hospital for further treatment.

Summary

Thirty years of clinical experience have shown that comprehensive care for pregnant women who use opioids can positively affect the outcome for both women and their children. Pregnancy offers a window of opportunity for treatment providers to help patients presenting with opioid dependence. MMT linked with appropriate woman-focused care can help a patient focus on her pregnancy and begin to deal with her substance dependence.

TABLE 15-2:

Neonatal abstinence score sheet

DATE:			DAILY WEIGHT:	
SIGNS AND SYMPTOMS	SCORE	AM	PM	COMMENTS
Central nervous system disturbances				
Excessive high-pitched cry	2			
Continuous high-pitched cry	3			
Sleeps < 1 hour after feeding	3			
Sleeps < 2 hours after feeding	2			
Sleeps < 3 hours after feeding	1			
Hyperactive Moro reflex	2			
Markedly hyperactive Moro reflex	3			
Mild tremors disturbed	1			
Moderate–severe tremors disturbed	2			
Mild tremors undisturbed	3			
Moderate–severe tremors undisturbed	4			
Increased muscle tone	2			
Excoriation (specific area)	1			
Myoclonic jerks	3			
Generalized convulsions	5			
Metabolic, vasomotor and respiratory disturbances				
Sweating	1			
Fever 37.2 to 38.3 °C	1			
Fever 38.4 °C and higher	2			
Frequent yawning (> 3–4 times/interval)	1			
Mottling	1			

Continued on next page

TABLE 15-2: NEONATAL ABSTINENCE SCORE SHEET (continued)

SIGNS AND SYMPTOMS	SCORE	AM						PM						COMMENTS
Metabolic, vasomotor, and respiratory disturbances														
Nasal stuffiness	1													
Sneezing (> 3–4 times/interval)	1													
Nasal flaring	2													
Respiratory rate > 60/min.	1													
Respiratory rate > 60/min. With retractions	2													
Gastrointestinal disturbances														
Excessive sucking	1													
Poor feeding	2													
Regurgitation	2													
Projectile vomiting	3													
Loose stools	2													
Watery stools	3													
TOTAL SCORE														

Reproduced with permission from Finnegan, L.P., Kron, R.E., Connaughton, J.F. & Emich, J.P., A scoring system for evaluation and treatment of the neonatal abstinence syndrome: A new clinical and research tool. In *Basic and Therapeutic Aspects of Perinatal Pharmacology*, Eds. Morselli, P.L., Garattini, S. & Sereni, F., New York: Raven Press, 139–155, 1975.

References

Alford D.P., Compton, P. & Samet, J.H. (2006). Acute pain management for patients receiving maintenance methadone or buprenorphine therapy. *Annals of Internal Medicine, 144 (2),* 127–134.

Anyaegbunam, A., Tran, T., Jadali, D., Randolph, G. & Mikhail, M.S. (1997). Assessment of fetal well-being in methadone-maintained pregnancies: Abnormal nonstress tests. *Gynecologic and Obstetric Investigation, 43* (1), 25–28.

Archie, C. (1998). Methadone in the management of narcotic addiction in pregnancy. *Current Opinion in Obstetrics and Gynecology, 10* (6), 435–440.

Archie, C.L., Lee, M.I, Sokol, R.J. & Norman, G. (1989). The effects of methadone treatment on the reactivity of the nonstress test. *Obstetrics and Gynecology, 74* (2), 254–255.

Bell, G.L. & Lau, K. (1995). Perinatal and neonatal issues of substance abuse. *Pediatric Clinics of North America, 42* (2), 261–281.

Berghella, V., Lim, P.J., Hill, M.K., Cherpes, J., Chennat, J. & Kaltenbach, K. (2003). Maternal methadone dose and neonatal withdrawal. *American Journal of Obstetrics and Gynecology, 189,* 312–317.

Blinick, G., Inturrisi, C.E., Jerez, E. & Wallach, R.C. (1974). Amniotic fluid methadone in women maintained on methadone. *Mount Sinai Journal of Medicine, 41,* 254–259.

Blinick, G., Wallach, R.C. & Jerez, E. (1969). Pregnancy in narcotics addicts treated by medical withdrawal. *American Journal of Obstetrics and Gynecology*, 105 (7), 997–1003.

Briggs, G.G., Freeman, R.K. & Yaffe, S.J. (2005). *Drugs in Pregnancy and Lactation* (7th ed.). Philadelphia: Lippincott Williams & Wilkins.

Cejtin, H., Mills, A. & Swift, E. (1996). Effect of methadone on the biophysical profile. *Journal of Reproductive Medicine, 15* (3), 819–822.

Chang, G., Carroll, K.M., Behr, H.M. & Kosten, T.R. (1992). Improving treatment outcome in pregnant opiate-dependent women. *Journal of Substance Abuse Treatment, 9* (4), 327–330.

Chasnoff, I.J., Hatcher, R. & Burns, W.J. (1982). Polydrug- and methadone-addicted newborns: A continuum of impairment? *Pediatrics, 70,* 210–213.

College of Physicians and Surgeons of Ontario. (2005). *Methadone Maintenance Guidelines.* Toronto: Author.

Connaughton, J.F., Reeser, D., Schut, J. & Finnegan, L.P. (1977). Perinatal addiction: Outcome and management. *American Journal of Obstetrics and Gynecology, 129,* 679–686.

Connor, E.M., Sperling, R.S., Gelber, R., Kiselev, P., Scott, G., O'Sullivan, M.J., et al., (1994). Reduction of maternal-infant transmission of human immunodeficiency virus type 1 with zidovudine treatment. *New England Journal of Medicine, 331,* 1173–1180.

Currie, J.C. (2001). *Best Practices Treatment and Rehabilitation for Women with Substance Use Problems.* Ottawa, ON: Health Canada.

Dashe, J.S., Jackson, G.L., Olscher, D.A., Zane, E.H. & Wendel, G.D. Jr. (1998). Opioid detoxification in pregnancy. *Obstetrics and Gynecology, 92* (5), 854–858.

Dashe, J.S., Sheffield, J.S., Olscher, D.A., Todd, S.J., Jackson, G.L. & Wendel, G.D. (2002). Relationship between maternal methadone dosage and neonatal withdrawal. *Obstetrics and Gynecology, 100,* 1244–1249.

DePetrillo, P.B. & Rice, J-M. (1995). Methadone dosing and pregnancy: Impact on program compliance. *International Journal of the Addictions, 30* (2), 207–217.

Doberczak, T.M., Kandall, S.R. & Friedmann, P. (1993). Relationship between maternal methadone dosage, maternal-neonatal methadone levels, and neonatal withdrawal. *Obstetrics and Gynecology, 81* (6), 936–40.

Doberczak, T.M., Kandall, S.R. & Wilets, I. (1991). Neonatal opiate abstinence syndrome in term and preterm infants. *The Journal of Pediatrics, 118* (6), 933–937.

Drozdick, J., Berghella, V., Hill, M.K. & Kaltenbach, K. (2002). Methadone trough levels in pregnancy. *American Journal of Obstetrics and Gynecology, 187,* 1184–1188.

Edelin, K.C., Gurganious, L., Golar, K., Oellerich, D., Kyei-Aboagye, K. & Hamid, M.A. (1988). Methadone maintenance in pregnancy: Consequences to care and outcome. *Obstetrics and Gynecology, 71* (3), 399–404.

Fajemirokun-Odudeyi, O., Sinha, C., Tutty, S., Pairaudeau, P., Armstrong, D., Phillips, T. et al. (2006). Pregnancy outcome in women who use opiates. *European Journal of Obstetrics and Gynecology and Reproductive Biology, 126,* 170–175.

Finnegan, L.P. (1975). A scoring system for evaluation and treatment of the neonatal abstinence syndrome: A new clinical and research tool. In P.L. Morselli, S. Garattini & F. Sereni (Eds.), *Basic and Therapeutic Aspects of Perinatal Pharmacology.* New York: Raven Press.

Finnegan, L.P. (1978). Management of pregnant drug-dependent women. *Annals of the New York Academy of Sciences, 311* (1), 135–146.

Finnegan, L.P. (Ed.). (1979). *Drug Dependence in Pregnancy: Clinical Management of Mother and Child.* NIDA Research Monograph. Rockville, MD: U.S. Department of Health, Education and Welfare.

Finnegan, L.P. (1983). Clinical perinatal and development effects of methadone. In J.R. Cooper, F. Altman, B.S. Brown & D. Czechowicz (Eds.), *Research on the Treatment of Narcotic Addiction: State of the Art.* Rockville, MD: National Institute on Drug Abuse. U.S. Department of Health and Human Services.

Finnegan, L.P. (1986). Neonatal abstinence syndrome: Assessment and pharmacotherapy. In Rubatelli F.F. and Granatt, B. (Eds.), *Neonatal Therapy: An Update.* Elsevier Sciences Publishers B.V.

Finnegan, L.P. (1991). Treatment issues for opioid-dependent women during the perinatal period. *Journal of Psychoactive Drugs, 23* (2), 191–201.

Finnegan, L.P. & Kaltenbach, K. (1992). Neonatal abstinence syndrome. In R.A. Hoekelman & N.M. Nelson (Eds.), *Primary Pediatric Care* (2nd ed.). St. Louis, MO: Mosby Yearbook Inc.

Finnegan, L.P., Kron, R.E., Connaughton, J.F. & Emich, J.P. (1975). Assessment and treatment of abstinence in the infant of the drug-dependent mother. *International Journal of Clinical Pharmacology, 12* (1/2), 19–32.

Fricker, H.S. & Segal, S. (1978). Narcotic addiction, pregnancy and the newborn. *American Journal of Diseases of Children, 132,* 360–366.

Giles, W., Patterson, T., Sanders, F., Batey, R., Thomas, D. & Collins, J. (1989). Outpatient methadone programme for pregnant heroin using women. *Australian and New Zealand Journal of Obstetrics and Gynaecology, 29* (3 Part 1), 225–229.

Gill, A.C., Oei, J., Lewis, N.L., Younan, N., Kennedy, I. & Lui, K. (2003). Strabismus in infants of opiate-dependent mothers. *Acta Paediatrica, 92* (3), 379–385.

Glatstein, M.M., Garcia-Bournissen, F., Finkelstein, Y. & Koren, G. (2008). Methadone exposure during lactation. *Canadian Family Physician, 54,* 1689–1690.

Hans, S.L. (1989). Developmental consequences of prenatal exposure to methadone. *Annals of the New York Academy of Sciences, 562,* 195–207.

Hoegerman, G. & Schnoll, S. (1991). Narcotic use in pregnancy. *Clinics in Perinatology, 18* (1), 51–76.

Hulse, G.K., Milne, E., English, D.R. & Holman, C.D.J. (1997). The relationship between maternal use of heroin and methadone and infant birth weight. *Addiction, 92* (11), 1571–1579.

Hulse, G.K., Milne, E., English, D.R. & Holman, C.D. (1998). Assessing the relationship between maternal opiate use and neonatal mortality. *Addiction, 93* (7), 1033–1042.

Hunt, R.W., Tzioumi, D., Collins, E. & Jeffery, H.E. (2008). Adverse neurodevelopmental outcome in infants exposed to opiate in-utero. *Early Human Development, 84,* 29–35.

Jansson, L.M., Dipietro, J.A., Velez, M., Elko, A., Knauer, H. & Kivlighan, K.T. (2009). Maternal methadone dosing schedule and fetal neurobehaviour. *The Journal of Maternal-Fetal and Neonatal Medicine, 22* (1), 29–35.

Jansson, L.M., Velez, M. & Harrow, C. (2004). Methadone maintenance and lactation: A review of the literature and current management guidelines. *Journal of Human Lactation, 20,* 62–71.

Jarvis, M.A.E. & Schnoll, S.H. (1994). Methadone treatment during pregnancy. *Journal of Psychoactive Drugs, 26* (2), 155–161.

Jarvis, M.A.E., Wu-Pong, S., Kniseley, J.S. & Schnoll, S.H. (1999). Alterations in methadone metabolism during late pregnancy. *Journal of Addictive Diseases, 18* (4), 51–59.

Jones, H.E., O'Grady, K.E., Malfi, D. & Tuten, M. (2008). Methadone maintenance vs. methadone taper during pregnancy: Maternal and neonatal outcomes. *American Journal on Addictions, 17,* 372–386.

Kaltenbach, K. & Comfort, M.L. (1997). Methadone maintenance of greater than 80 mg during pregnancy. *NIDA Research Monograph, 174,* 128.

Kaltenbach, K. & Finnegan, L.P. (1986). Neonatal abstinence syndrome, pharmacotherapy and developmental outcome. *Neurotoxicology and Teratology, 8,* 353–355.

Kaltenbach, K. & Finnegan, L.P. (1987). Perinatal and developmental outcome of infants exposed to methadone in utero. *Neurotoxicology and Teratology, 9* (4), 311–313.

Kaltenbach, K. & Finnegan, L.P. (1992). Methadone maintenance during pregnancy: Implications for perinatal and developmental outcome. In T.B. Sonderegger (Ed.), *Perinatal Substance Abuse: Research Findings and Clinical Implications.* Baltimore, MD: Johns Hopkins University Press.

Kaltenbach, K., Berghella, V. & Finnegan, L. (1998). Opioid dependence during pregnancy: Effects and management. *Obstetrics and Gynecology Clinics of North America, 25* (1), 139–151.

Kandall, S.R., Albin, S., Gartner, L.M., Lee, K.S., Eidelman, A. & Lowinson, J. (1977). The narcotic-dependent mother: Fetal and neonatal consequences. *Early Human Development, 1* (2), 159–169.

Kandall, S.R., Albin, S., Lowinson, J., Berle, B., Eidelman, A.I. & Gartner, L.M. (1976). Differential effects of maternal heroin and methadone use on birthweight. *Pediatrics, 58* (5), 681–685.

Kandall, S.R., Doberczak, T.M., Jantunen, M. & Stein, J. (1999). The methadone-maintained pregnancy. *Clinics in Perinatology, 26* (1), 173–183.

Levine, A. & Rebarber, A. (1995). Methadone maintenance treatment the nonstress test. *Journal of Perinatology, 15* (3), 229–231.

Lifschitz, M.H., Wilson, G.S., Smith, E.O. & Desmond, M. (1985). Factors affecting head growth and intellectual function in children of drug addicts. *Pediatrics, 75,* 269–274.

Liston, R., Sawchuck, D. & Young, D. (2007). Fetal health surveillance: antepartum and intrapartum consensus guideline. *Journal of Obstetrics and Gynaecology Canada, 197,* S1–S56.

Little, B.B., Snell, L.M., Klein, V.R., Gilstrap, L.C., Knoll, K.A. & Breckenridge, J.D. (1990). Maternal and fetal effects of heroin addiction during pregnancy. *Journal of Reproductive Medicine, 35* (2), 159–162.

Luty, J., Nikolaou, V. & Bearn, J. (2003). Is opiate detoxification unsafe in pregnancy? *Journal of Substance Abuse Treatment, 24,* 363–367.

Maas, U., Kattner, E., Weingart-Jesse, B., Schäfer, A. & Obladen, M. (1990). Infrequent neonatal opiate withdrawal following maternal methadone detoxification during pregnancy. *Journal of Perinatal Medicine, 18,* 111–118.

McCarthy, J.J., Leamon, M.H., Parr, M.S. & Anania, B. (2005). High-dose methadone maintenance in pregnancy: Maternal and neonatal outcomes. *American Journal of Obstetrics and Gynecology, 193*, 606–610.

Mehta, V. & Langford, R.M. (2006). Acute pain management for opioid dependent patients. *Anaesthesia, 61*, 269–276.

Nelson, L.B., Ehrlich, S., Calhoun, J.H., Matteucci, T. & Finnegan, L.P. (1987). Occurrence of strabismus in infants born to drug-dependent women. *American Journal of Diseases of Children, 141*, 175–178.

Pond, S.M., Kreek, M.J., Tong, T.G., Raghunath, J. & Benowitz, N.L. (1985). Altered methadone pharmacokinetics in methadone-maintained pregnant women. *Journal of Pharmacology and Experimental Therapeutics, 233* (1), 1–6.

Reisine, T. & Pasternak, G. (1996). Opioid analgesics and antagonists. In J.G. Hardman & L.E. Limbird (Eds.), *Goodman & Gilman's The Pharmacological Basis of Therapeutics*, Toronto: McGraw-Hill.

Rementeria, J.L. & Nunag, N.N. (1973). Narcotic withdrawal in pregnancy: Stillbirth incidence with a case report. *American Journal of Obstetrics & Gynecology, 116* (3), 1152–1156.

Santen, R.J., Sofsky, J., Bilic, N. & Lippert, R. (1975). Mechanism of action of narcotics in the production of menstrual dysfunction in women. *Fertility and Sterility, 26* (6), 538–548.

Scimeca, M.M., Savage, S.R., Portenoy, R. & Lowinson, J. (2000). Treatment of pain in methadone-maintained patients. *The Mount Sinai Journal of Medicine, 67* (5 & 6), 412–422.

Stern, R. (1966). The pregnant addict. *American Journal of Obstetrics and Gynecology, 94* (2), 253–257.

Stimmel, B., Goldberg, J., Reisman, A., Murphy, R.J. & Teets, K. (1983). Fetal outcome in narcotic-dependent women: The importance of the type of maternal narcotic used. *American Journal of Drug and Alcohol Abuse, 9* (4), 383–395.

Swift, R.M., Dudley, M., DePetrillo, P., Camara, P. & Griffiths, W. (1989). Altered methadone pharmacokinetics in pregnancy: Implications for dosing. *Journal of Substance Abuse, 1* (4), 453–460.

Vance, J.C., Chant, D.C., Tudehope, D.I., Gray, P.H. & Hayes, A.J. (1997). Infants born to narcotic dependent mothers: Physical growth patterns in the first 12 months of life. *Journal of Paediatrics and Child Health, 33* (6), 504–508.

Vucinovic, M., Roje, D., Vucinovic, Z., Capkun, V., Bucat, M. & Banovic, I. (2008). Maternal and neonatal effects of substance abuse during pregnancy: Our ten-year experience. *Yonsei Medical Journal, 49* (5), 705–713.

Wilson, G.S., Desmond, M.M. & Wait, R.B. (1981). Follow-up of methadone-treated and untreated narcotic-dependent women and their infants: Health, developmental, and social implications. *Journal of Pediatrics, 98* (5), 716–722.

Wittmann, B.K. & Segal, S. (1991). A comparison of the effects of single- and split-dose methadone administration on the fetus: Ultrasound evaluation. *International Journal of Addictions, 26* (2), 213–218.

Wolff, K., Boys, A., Rostami-Hodjegan, A., Hay, A. & Raistrick D. (2005). Changes to methadone clearance during pregnancy. *European Journal of Clinical Pharmacology, 61*, 763–768.

Wong, T. & Lee, S.S. (2006). Hepatitis C: A review for primary care physicians. *Canadian Medical Association Journal, 174* (5), 649–659.

Wunsch, M., Stanard, V. & Schnoll, S. (2003). Treatment of pain in pregnancy. *Clinical Journal of Pain, 19* (3), 148–155.

Zelson, C., Lee, S.J. & Casalino, M. (1973). Neonatal narcotic addiction: Comparative effects of maternal intake of heroin and methadone. *New England Journal of Medicine, 289* (23), 1216–1220.

Zuspan, F.P., Gumpel, J.A., Mejia-Zelaya, A., Madden J. & Davis, R. (1975). Fetal stress from methadone withdrawal. *American Journal of Obstetrics and Gynecology, 122* (1), 43–46.

CHAPTER 16

MMT and special-needs populations

This chapter discusses the particular challenges of maintaining patients on methadone in several special contexts, such as hospitalization or incarceration. It also provides a brief overview of considerations respecting MMT for older adults and youth.

Protocol for hospitalized methadone patients

CONTINUITY OF CARE

There is rarely a clinical indication for discontinuing methadone in MMT patients who need to be hospitalized, and such discontinuation can have serious medical consequences (Freidman et al., 2003).

General hospitals should have methadone in their formulary. If the hospital in question does not, the patient should provide his or her own carry bottles if they are available. Only unopened, properly labelled carry bottles should be used.

A physician can obtain a temporary methadone licence from the Office of Controlled Substances, valid only while the patient is in hospital. However, in our experience it is safer if a physician experienced with methadone prescribes it. If there is no such physician on staff, the hospital should find a licensed physician in the community.

Emergency department

When patients are held in the emergency department for more than 24 hours after their last methadone dose, follow the protocol described below.

DOSAGE

The patient's community pharmacy should be contacted to verify the correct dosage, the date and time the last dose was dispensed, the number of carries the patient has been given, and the patient's attendance record at the pharmacy (number of days missed per week or month). The patient should be asked if any carry doses were taken as prescribed and, if possible, should be requested to show their carry bottles to the nurse. The methadone prescription at the patient's regular pharmacy should be cancelled for the duration of the patient's hospital stay.

If it is impossible to verify the dosage because the physician cannot be reached and the pharmacy is closed, the patient may receive a long-acting oral opioid such as MS Contin 30 mg tid, or methadone at the starting dose (20 to 30 mg). This will not fully relieve withdrawal symptoms, but should keep the patient relatively comfortable until the dose can be verified.

Dosage adjustment in hospital

Under most circumstances, patients will continue on their regular dose while in hospital; however, a patient on a stable methadone dose is at increased risk for methadone toxicity if he or she:

- is given benzodiazepines or other sedating drugs
- has a decreased level of consciousness
- has an acute respiratory illness such as pneumonia
- has missed three or more doses prior to hospitalization, or
- is on a quinolone antibiotic or other medication that inhibits methadone metabolism.

In any of the above cases, the physician should order "hold methadone dose if drowsy" and assess the patient daily for signs of methadone toxicity. If the physician feels the patient is at substantial risk for methadone toxicity because of any of the above circumstances, the dose should be decreased by 20 to 40 per cent, with a rapid dose increase once the danger has passed.

NPO PATIENTS

Patients who cannot have the orange drink that methadone is usually dispensed with can take it in water. If a patient is unable to take any oral medications (designated NPO) withdrawal can be lessened with scheduled doses of parenteral morphine or hydromorphone. Use of peripheral and central lines should be limited in unstable patients if possible.

INPATIENT ORDERS

A physician not authorized to prescribe methadone may obtain emergency authorization by placing a telephone call to the Office of Controlled Substances, Health Canada. As with an outpatient prescription, any inpatient order should specify the dose and the start and end date. The order should also specify that the dose must be witnessed. The prescribing physician should ask to be informed if the patient receives new medications, particularly sedating medications or those that interfere with methadone metabolism.

Methadone kept in a hospital should be stored in a locked narcotic cupboard and dispensed under the supervision of a nurse.

DISCHARGE

The patient may be given the morning methadone dose on the day of discharge and told to contact his or her regular prescribing physician immediately. The hospital physician should also contact the methadone prescriber directly with any relevant information. For example, if the patient was admitted for a suicide attempt, the methadone physician will need to reassess the patient's take-home dose privileges. If the patient was discharged with a prescription for benzodiazepines or quinolone antibiotics, the physician may need to readjust the methadone dose.

INPATIENT INITIATION OF METHADONE

Methadone treatment can be initiated in a hospital setting (see Table 16–1). The starting dose is usually 10 to 20 mg, followed by two 5 mg prn doses. If these prn doses are used over the next two days, on the third morning the dose should be increased by 5 to 10 mg, followed by two 5 mg prn doses. With this protocol, a daily dose of 50 mg may be achieved within a week.

Vigilance is required from hospital staff, as methadone overdose deaths have occurred even in an inpatient setting. An experienced methadone physician should prescribe the methadone, and nurses should be advised to carefully monitor the patient and hold the dose if he or she becomes drowsy. The use of benzodiazepines and other sedating drugs should be minimized. Extreme caution should be used in initiating methadone treatment in a patient with an acute respiratory illness or altered level of consciousness from any cause.

TABLE 16–1

Inpatient intiation of methadone protocol

	REGULAR DOSE	PRN DOSE
Day 1 and day 2	10–20 mg	5 mg, maximum 2x in 24 hours
Day 3 and day 4	10–30 mg	5 mg, maximum 2x in 24 hours
Day 5 and day 6	10–40 mg	
Day 7	10–50 mg	

NON-MEDICAL TREATMENT SETTINGS

MMT can usually be continued in withdrawal management centres, shelters and other non-medical treatment facilities. The prescriber should contact the agency to locate a nearby pharmacy that dispenses methadone, and the agency should arrange a time for the patient to receive daily dispensing from the pharmacy. The agency should not dispense methadone on site.

Management of MMT in correctional facilities

JURISDICTION AND POLICY ISSUES

In Canada, the constitutional authority for the judicial system is divided between the federal and provincial governments. If people are sentenced to two or more years, they are usually sent to a federal prison. In Ontario, the Ministry of Community Safety and Correctional Services has jurisdiction over the following offenders: adults over the age of 18 who have been sentenced to imprisonment for less than two years and/or probation for up to three years, or have received conditional sentences of up to two years less a day. The ministry also has jurisdiction over those adult offenders on parole, on remand, or awaiting trial or sentencing; adults held for immigration hearings or deportation; and those offenders awaiting transfer to federal institutions to serve sentences of two years or more.

Although it is not legal to use drugs in correctional facilities in Canada, injection drug use is quite prevalent in this setting (Choopanya et al., 2002). Moreover, since injection paraphernalia is in short supply, sharing among inmates is common, including both HIV-positive and HIV-negative inmates (Wood, Li et al., 2005). This sharing leads to high rates of transmission of infectious diseases such as HIV and hepatitis C (Choopanya et al., 2002; Wood, Kerr et al., 2005; Clarke et al., 2001; Baillargeon et al., 1999; Cotton-Oldenburg et al., 1999).

Methadone is recommended for incarcerated people who meet the criteria for opioid dependence (Dolan et al., 1998). Prescribing methadone for such patients may reduce disease transmission among inmates by reducing needle sharing. Moreover, patients who are in MMT programs and find themselves incarcerated should have continuity of treatment to maintain the health benefits derived from methadone. Opioid-dependent inmates who are being released from jail are also good candidates for MMT if they have not been offered MMT while in jail (Rich, McKenzie et al., 2005).

The biggest concern with this population is the risk of opioid overdose and associated mortality that can occur in abstinent inmates who relapse immediately upon their release from jail (Harding-Pink, 1990; Seal et al., 2001). Moreover, inmates have reported diversion of methadone in Canadian jails, sometimes with fatal consequences. The family of one woman who died of a methadone overdose while in jail launched a lawsuit against the federal and provincial government (CBC News, 2005).

Appropriate policies are needed in correctional facilities to ensure that patients who require methadone receive it according to best practices and that diversion is minimized to prevent overdoses in other inmates. In addition, appropriate linkages between community providers of MMT and correctional facilities need to be established to prevent the interruption of MMT for patients who become incarcerated during the course of treatment. Further, opioid-dependent individuals being released from jails should be connected with methadone providers as soon as possible (Rich, McKenzie et al., 2005).

Policies regarding MMT in federal prisons are outlined in the document *Correctional Service of Canada: Specific Guidelines for Methadone Maintenance Treatment*, 2003.

PRESCRIBING METHADONE TO NEW INMATES

Dosing on admission

All inmates who are enrolled in MMT should be provided methadone when it is due from the time of their admission—there should be no interruption in their treatment.

Before prescribing methadone, the prison physician should obtain the name and address of the MMT physician and pharmacy in the community to confirm the following information:

- the amount and time of administration of the last observed dose

- whether or not the patient has had any take-home doses
- other relevant history, such as concomitant substance use, other prescriptions and comorbid medical and psychiatric problems.

If the patient's existing dose of methadone and pattern of ingestion cannot be determined, the attending prison physician may prescribe up to and including 30 mg of methadone per day until the dose can be confirmed.

It is important to receive informed and signed consent from the inmate and fax a copy to the MMT physician.

If, in the judgment of the prison physician, the dose requires adjustment, frequent assessment of the patient is recommended. Sedating drugs such as benzodiazepines should be avoided or tapered wherever possible. Methadone may be given in divided doses if there is a concern about the level of tolerance, although this approach may not be feasible within a prison for logistical reasons.

If a physician in the community is contacted by a prison nurse about a patient of the physician's in a correctional facility, with a request to prescribe and continue medication, the CPSO's guidelines allow for a faxed prescription to be sent to the prison pharmacy until the prison physician assumes care for the patient. In the case of methadone, it is important to have the prison nurse confirm the inmate's level of alertness and use of concomitant medications, as well as the time the last dose was administered, before the prescription is faxed over. If a dose has been missed for three or more days, this should trigger an alert that the usual prescribed dose needs to be reduced until the inmate can be assessed by the attending prison physician.

Take-home doses in patient's possession at time of admission

If a patient arrives at a correctional facility with bottles of methadone, these should be disposed of appropriately. It is impossible to be certain of the contents of the bottle. Under no circumstances should an inmate be allowed to self-administer methadone, even if the detention will be only for a short while. Inmates should surrender any carry doses they have, and should be reassured that they will be given their prescribed dose by prison health staff. In Canada, there have been overdose deaths in patients serving weekend sentences (also known as intermittent sentences) who brought their own methadone to the facility.

INITIATING METHADONE IN PRISON POPULATIONS

Assessment

Some prison authorities feel that prisoners facing a long sentence have no need of methadone but should instead be withdrawn from all opioids (Rich, Boutwell et al., 2005). However, due to the high rates of drug use and disease transmission in prisons, it may be appropriate to commence MMT for dependent patients within a correctional facility (Kinlock et al., 2002; Heimer et al., 2005).

Prisons should make it a priority to initiate MMT for qualifying inmates who are HIV-positive, HCV- or HBV-positive or pregnant.

One particular challenge for prison physicians is assessing the actuality of opioid dependence in inmates. Sometimes a patient provides a compelling story of opioid dependence, but his or her urine drug screen is negative (unless the inmate used while in prison). There may be no evidence of opioid withdrawal in an inmate who is seen more than a week after admission to the prison. Whenever feasible, corroborating data regarding the patient's history of opioid use should be obtained from other sources. It is also possible to conduct hair analysis to confirm long-term opioid use, but this test is not readily available within prison laboratories.

If there is a doubt about the patient's actually having used opioids, it is important to start with a very low dose of methadone (i.e., 5 mg) and to reassess the patient within three to five days. Since the risk of overdose is the highest in the first two weeks of MMT, ongoing observation by prison staff is recommended. It is better to initiate MMT for new inmates early in the week so that medical staff can observe the inmate more closely. Methadone should not be given before bedtime, and other sedating drugs should be avoided.

Practical considerations

Standard of care

Incarcerated patients have the right to the same standard of care as the rest of the population. Therefore, as in other instances, multidisciplinary care is recommended, and confidentiality should be maintained. A prison-based MMT program requires clear communication among correctional staff, health care providers and inmates enrolled in the program. All stakeholders should be clear about the following information:

- the expectations of each member of the care provision team
- the times and procedures for the administration of methadone
- the policies on the use of urine drug screening
- the schedule of appointments with the prison physician and counsellors.

In general, as in other populations, vomited doses of methadone should be replaced, with rare exceptions (see Table 15-1 on page 138 for a schedule for replacement doses). No inmates or non-medical prison staff should have access to the methadone, which must be stored in a locked refrigerator within a secured medication room. A treatment agreement should be signed with each patient and made part of his or her medical record.

CPSO reporting requirements

In Ontario, all inmates initiated on MMT need to be registered with the College of Physicians and Surgeons of Ontario (CPSO).

The CPSO requires initiation and cessation forms for any incarcerated patient given MMT. In cases of intermittent detention, such as weekend sentencing, the community physician and the prison staff should make arrangements for observed ingestion. No transfer of care is necessary.

Observed administration

All methadone should be dispensed and consumed under direct observation to minimize the risk of diversion.

Procedures should be in place, and carefully followed, to minimize medication errors. These include using photo identification, cross-checking doses and routinizing protocols. Records should be kept of the timing and amount of each dose administered for each inmate. To minimize the risk of diversion, inmates given methadone should be observed and segregated from other inmates for at least 20 to 30 minutes after each dose, during which time they should not be allowed to be alone even to visit the washroom. Each inmate should be asked to consume at least 8 oz. of fluid both before and after the methadone is administered, and the methadone should be diluted in an orange drink per standard guidelines. The inmate's mouth should be inspected for wads of cloth before and after the dose is consumed to make sure the methadone is not diverted.

Take-home doses and weekend passes

Take-home doses are not recommended for incarcerated patients who are released on weekend passes. Arrangements for observed ingestion should be made in a community pharmacy.

Urine drug screening

Urine drug screening in a prison-based MMT program should be treated as part of the medical protocol—it should not be available to prison staff for punitive purposes. The prison physician should use urine drug screening to guide response to treatment, and its purpose should be clearly communicated to patients.

Overdose

All inmates given methadone should be observed for excess sedation. Any inmate who is suspected of taking methadone and is showing early signs of overdose should be managed in an emergency room. It is not safe or appropriate to let an inmate "sleep it off" and possibly overdose.

Transfer of care upon discharge

If the release date for an inmate is known, arrangements for the transfer of his or her care should be made in advance. The attending prison physician should make arrangements for daily observed methadone dispensing in a community pharmacy to overlap with the first appointment with the methadone-prescribing physician in the community. It is also important that the prison fax appropriate cessation forms to the CPSO, and send, with the patient's consent, any pertinent health information to the new physician.

Prescriptions should not be handed over to the inmate, and it is not recommended that take-home doses be granted to an inmate being released. Clear communication between the two physicians is important to avoid the risk of double-dosing. If the patient is going to a community without access to MMT, it is important to initiate and complete a taper off methadone before discharge, and to educate the patient about the high risk of overdose in the case of relapse. If the patient is willing to take naltrexone, it should be initiated at least 10 days after the last dose of methadone to avoid precipitating withdrawal.

Unexpected release

Sometimes, an inmate appears in court and is unexpectedly released directly to the community. It is therefore important to educate patient inmates about the protocols to follow if they are released in such a manner.

They should be advised to carry contact information for the medical staff at the correctional facility whenever they make a court appearance if there is even a remote possibility they may be released or transferred to another facility.

Upon release, a patient should contact the prison medical staff immediately to make arrangements for daily-observed methadone ingestion in a community pharmacy. He or she should be advised to contact a methadone-prescribing physician for admission to an appropriate program. In Ontario, the CPSO Methadone Program (416 967-2661) can provide a list of prescribing physicians, and the Ontario College of Pharmacists (416 962-4861) can provide a list of local pharmacies that dispense methadone.

MMT programs in correctional facilities complement community-based programs and have great potential for improving the health of inmates who are opioid dependent.

Other special populations

OLDER ADULTS

Methadone treatment is not contraindicated in elderly patients, but clinicians should consider a lower initial dose (5 to 10 mg), with slow and careful titration, for this population. The titration might need to be done in a supervised setting if the patient is medically ill or on multiple medications.

YOUTH

Before diagnosing opioid dependence in a young person, the physician should obtain corroborating information if possible. There have been case reports of youth who were not opioid dependent attempting to obtain prescriptions for methadone for its euphoric effects. Some therapists advocate that youth in MMT should be kept away from older methadone clients and should receive youth-specific treatment if possible.

Youth and adults with a short history of opioid dependence may benefit from a slow taper off methadone, and they may be good candidates for buprenorphine treatment.

References

Baillargeon, J., Borucki, M., Williamson, J. & Dunn, K. (1999). Determinants of HIV-related survival among Texas prison inmates. *AIDS Patient Care and STDs 13*, 355–361.

CBC News. (2005). *Family launches lawsuit over methadone death.* Available at: www.cbc.ca/canada/saskatchewan/story/2005/01/18/keepness-sonia050118.html.

Choopanya, K., Des Jarlais, D.C., Vanichseni, S., Kitayaporn, D., Mock, P.A., Raktham, S. et al. (2002). Incarceration and risk for HIV infection among injection drug users in Bangkok. *Journal of Acquired Immune Deficiency Syndromes, 29*, 86–94.

Clarke, J.G., Stein, M.D., Hanna, L., Sobota, M. & Rich, J.D. (2001). Active and former injection drug users report of HIV risk behaviors during periods of incarceration. *Substance Abuse, 22*, 209–216.

Correctional Service of Canada. (2003). *Specific Guidelines for Methadone Maintenance Treatment.* Ottawa: Author. Available at www.csc-scc.gc.ca/text/pblct/methadone/index-eng.shtml.

Cotton-Oldenburg, N.U., Jordan, B.K., Martin, S.L. & Sadowski, L.S. (1999). Voluntary HIV testing in prison: Do women inmates at high risk for HIV accept HIV testing? *AIDS Education and Prevention, 11*, 28–37.

Dolan, K.A., Wodak, A.D. & Hall, W.D. (1998). Methadone maintenance treatment reduces heroin injection in New South Wales prisons. *Drug and Alcohol Review, 17,* 153–158.

Friedman, R., Kamel, I., Perez, C. & Hamada, A. (2003). Severe intraoperative hypertension and opioid-resistant postoperative pain in a methadone-treated patient. *Journal of Pain, 4* (5), 289–290.

Harding-Pink, D. (1990). Mortality following release from prison. *Medicine, Science, and the Law, 30*, 12–16.

Heimer, R., Catania, H., Newman, R.G., Zambrano, J., Brunet, A. & Ortiz, A.M. (2005). Methadone maintenance in prison: Evaluation of a pilot program in Puerto Rico. *Drug and Alcohol Dependence, 83* (2), 122–129.

Kinlock, T.W., Battjes, R.J. & Schwartz, R.P. (2002). A novel opioid maintenance program for prisoners: Preliminary findings. *Journal of Substance Abuse Treatment, 22,* 141–147.

Rich, J.D., Boutwell, A.E., Shield, D.C., Key, R.G., McKenzie, M., Clarke, J.G. et al. (2005). Attitudes and practices regarding the use of methadone in US state and federal prisons. *Journal of Urban Health, 82*, 411–419.

Rich, J.D., McKenzie, M., Shield, D.C., Wolf, F.A., Key, R.G., Poshkus, M. et al. (2005). Linkage with methadone treatment upon release from incarceration: a promising opportunity. *Journal of Addictive Diseases, 24*, 49–59.

Seal, K.H., Kral, A.H., Gee, L., Moore, L.D., Bluenthal, R.N., Lorvick, J. et al. (2001). Predictors and prevention of nonfatal overdose among street-recruited injection heroin users in the San Francisco Bay Area, 1998–1999. *American Journal of Public Health, 91*, 1842–1846.

Wood, E., Kerr, T., Stoltz, J., Qui, Z., Zhang, R., Montaner, J.S.G. et al. (2005). Prevalence and correlates of hepatitis C infection among users of North America's first medically supervised safer injection facility. *Public Health 119,* 1111–1115.

Wood, E., Li, K., Small, W., Montaner, J.S., Schechter, M.T. & Kerr, T. (2005). Recent incarceration independently associated with syringe sharing by injection drug users. *Public Health Reports, 120*, 150–156.

CHAPTER 17

Methadone and driving

This chapter discusses the issues and evidence relating to the safety of MMT patients and driving. It suggests criteria for reporting impaired driving to provincial authorities and outlines some suggested protocols.

Prevalence and evidence

Methadone patients do not appear to have a higher rate of accidents or traffic charges than the general population (Maddux et al., 1977). Most methadone patients who have been involved in motor vehicle accidents or charged with impaired driving have shown toxicological evidence of having used other drugs, including alcohol, benzodiazepines, cannabis, cocaine or other opioids (Augsburger et al., 1997; Musshoff et al., 2003).

Experimental studies regarding the safety of driving while on methadone have produced conflicting results. In two studies, the majority of methadone patients had reduced performance on driving tests (Staak et al., 1993; Dittert et al., 1999). Patients in these studies who showed no evidence of other drug use (such as cannabis or alcohol) performed better than those who were using other drugs and performed almost, but not quite, as well as the control group (Hauri-Bionda et al., 1998). The methadone dose was not correlated with performance in these studies. Two studies comparing the driving skills of methadone and buprenorphine patients have had conflicting results (Lenne et al., 2003; Schindler et al., 2004), although a randomized trial found that patients assigned to the buprenorphine group had better cognitive and psychomotor performance than patients in the methadone group. There were no differences at baseline (Soyka et al., 2005).

Other opioids do not appear to impair driving ability when used in moderate, stable doses (Byas-Smith et al., 2005). However, the studies that support this finding have not examined the impact on cognitive or driving performance of poorly controlled pain and anxiety, high doses of opioids, or combination pharmacotherapy (opioids and TCAs, anticonvulsants or benzodiazepines).

Overall, there is fair evidence that methadone impairs driving ability when combined with other psychoactive drugs (alcohol, cannabis, benzodiazepines and cocaine). Some experimental studies have documented marginal decreases in driving performance from the use of methadone alone, but the clinical significance of these decreases is uncertain, as there is no epidemiological evidence that methadone used on its own is a risk factor for motor vehicle accidents. Other factors may impair performance in MMT patients, such as previous head injuries and personality factors.

Reporting to provincial authorities

The Ministry of Transportation of Ontario requires attending physicians to report any patient who has a medical condition that may impair his or her ability to operate a motor vehicle. The law does not allow for discretion on the part of the physician.

We suggest the following criteria (note that these opinions are those of the authors and do not carry legal weight):

- The patient regularly drives and uses benzodiazepines, cannabis, cocaine or alcohol during the day.
- The patient admits to using alcohol or other drugs and driving.
- A family member informs the physician that the patient is using drugs and driving.
- The patient drove to the physician's clinic while intoxicated.

- The patient regularly drives and has recently experienced a withdrawal seizure or drug/alcohol-induced seizure.
- The patient has a substance-related medical complication that may impair driving ability (e.g., alcohol-induced cerebellar ataxia or dementia).

ASSESSING INTOXICATION

If the patient drove to the clinic and the physician suspects intoxication, a clinical assessment should be performed. The physician should:

- take a quantitative history of alcohol and drug use for that day
- document slurred speech, nodding off, drowsiness, emotional lability or other signs of intoxication
- ask the patient to perform cerebellar tests (walking heel to toe, pointing finger to nose)
- order a blood alcohol content (BAC) test or urine drug screen, and inform the patient why (patients have the right to refuse)
- not permit the patient to drive, or even to leave the clinic with car keys (it may be necessary to call 911 if the patient refuses to hand over the keys).

INFORMING THE PATIENT OF A DECISION TO REPORT

If the physician decides that a report is appropriate, he or she should explain to the patient that:

- there is a legal obligation to make the report,
- the decision to suspend the licence is made by the authorities, and
- the patient has the right to appeal that decision.

Patients sometimes ask the physician to give them a chance to abstain and attend treatment before deciding to report them. However, trusting the patient to comply with instructions is not considered an adequate reason for failing to report.

AFTER A SUSPENSION

While patients are often angry about being reported, physicians can use the opportunity to advise them on the need for abstinence, counselling and treatment. Sometimes the embarrassment and inconvenience of a licence suspension are powerful motivators for change.

A patient's license is generally reinstated once the authorities have received confirmation from the physician that the patient has attended treatment and maintained abstinence or low-risk drinking for a specified number of months. Monthly patient visits are recommended.

At each visit, the physician should

- ask about drug or alcohol consumption,
- monitor with urine drug screens (and GGT and MCV if alcohol is an issue),
- with the patient's permission, ask a spouse/partner or close family member to corroborate the patient's reported substance use, and
- encourage the patient to attend aftercare.

Precautions regarding driving

There are some cases where reporting is not justified, but the physician may still want to take some precautions regarding driving and safety.

For several days after each methadone dose increase, patients should be encouraged not to drive for at least four to six hours after taking the dose. This is particularly important in the first few weeks of titration.

Patients who use a therapeutic dose of benzodiazepines at night do not necessarily need to be reported unless they use more than prescribed. Patients who are on daytime doses of benzodiazepines and need to drive regularly should have their doses reduced or tapered off completely. If they are unwilling to do so, the physician should consider making a report.

References

Augsburger, M. & Rivier, L. (1997). Drugs and alcohol among suspected impaired drivers in Canton de Vaud (Switzerland). *Forensic Science International, 85* (2), 95–104.

Byas-Smith, M.G., Chapman, S.L., Reed, B. & Cotsonis, G. (2005). The effect of opioids on driving and psychomotor performance in patients with chronic pain. *Clinical Journal of Pain, 21* (4), 345–352.

Dittert, S., Naber, D. & Soyka, M. (1999). Methadone substitution therapy and driving: Results of an experimental study. *Der Nervenarzt, 70* (5), 457–462.

Hauri-Bionda, R., Bar, W. & Friedrich-Koch, A. (1998). Driving fitness/driving capacity of patients treated with methadone. *Schweizerische Medizinische Wochenschrift, 128* (41), 1538–1547.

Lenne, M.G., Dietze, P., Rumbold, G.R., Redman, J.R. & Triggs, T.J. (2003). The effects of the opioid pharmacotherapies methadone, LAAM and buprenorphine, alone and in combination with alcohol, on simulated driving. *Drug and Alcohol Dependence, 72* (3), 271–278.

Maddux, J.F., Williams, T.R. & Ziegler, J.A. (1977). Driving records before and during methadone maintenance. *American Journal of Drug and Alcohol Abuse, 4* (1), 91–100.

Musshoff, F., Lachenmeier, D.W. & Madea, B. (2003). Methadone substitution: Medicolegal problems in Germany. *Forensic Science International, 133* (1–2), 118–124.

Schindler, S.D., Ortner, R., Peternell, A., Eder, H., Opgenoorth, E. & Fischer, G. (2004). Maintenance therapy with synthetic opioids and driving aptitude. *European Addiction Research, 10* (2), 80–87.

Soyka, M., Hock, B., Kagerer, S., Lehnert, R., Limmer, C. & Kuefner, H. (2005). Less impairment on one portion of a driving-relevant psychomotor battery in buprenorphine-maintained than in methadone-maintained patients: Results of a randomized clinical trial. *Journal of Clinical Psychopharmacology, 25* (5), 490–493.

Staak, M., Berghaus, G., Glazinski, R., Hoher, K., Joo, S. & Friedel, B. (1993). Empirical studies of automobile driving fitness of patients treated with methadone–substitution. *Blutalkohol, 30* (6), 321-333.

www.ingramcontent.com/pod-product-compliance
Ingram Content Group UK Ltd.
Pitfield, Milton Keynes, MK11 3LW, UK
UKHW051503290926
15471UKWH00008B/1378

9 781770 528925